THE ART OF

BABY-MAKING

THE ART OF
BABY-MAKING

THE HOLISTIC APPROACH
TO FERTILITY

GERAD KITE

Published in 2016 by
Short Books, Unit 316, ScreenWorks, 22 Highbury Grove,
London, N5 2ER

10 9 8 7 6 5 4 3 2 1

A CIP catalogue record for this book
is available from the British Library.

ISBN: 978-1-78072-278-8

Cover design by Andrew Smith

Printed at CPI Group (UK) Ltd, Croydon, CR0 4YY

To my parents
With all my love

CONTENTS

Introduction   9

Unexplained Infertility   18
    A Holistic Approach   23
    An Accidental Expert   29

The Nature of Balance   32
    A Philosophical Approach 38
    Finding Balance   41

The Five Elements   48
    Wood   48
    Fire   54
    Earth   58
    Metal   63
    Water   67

Spirit   73

Optimising Your Fertility   82
    Violating Natural Laws   85
    The Law of Midday-Midnight 91
    Men v Women   100
    Balance "With a Twist"   106

Relationships   112
    Bigger Relationships   122
    Love   130
    Sex   139
    The Importance of Orgasms 149

A Balanced Mind   154

    Being in the Moment   165

    If Only   168

    Faith   171

    Stop Trying   176

A Fresh Perspective   192

    Intention   196

    Gratitude   205

The Fertility "Business"   208

    Success   218

    The Gift   234

Tools For Balance   240

    Drinking Water   240

    Eating Breakfast   243

    True Rest   244

    The Pendulum   248

A Note on JR Worsley   250

Glossary   252

Introduction

Our love of babies and instinctive need to procreate are the most powerful driving forces of humanity. The desire to see the next generation flourish is hardwired into our DNA and even those of us who, for whatever reason, do not have children, depend on and enjoy what the next generation brings. In recent years, troubled by falling fertility rates, we humans have started to dabble in the baby-making business. Western medicine has decided that infertility is a modern problem in need of a modern solution. Yet, when it comes to baby-making we really are amateurs; nature has been doing this job since the beginning of time.

The Art of Baby-Making invites you to look at fertility and conception in a positive new light. This book is about *all* people, and not just those who want to have children. The issues surrounding this epidemic of infertility are far bigger than you might think. They're a reflection of the quality of life, not just of prospective parents but of humanity in general. As modern life provides for our every material need and technology brings the world directly into our homes, our creativity and discovery of self are starting to be seriously compromised. We are less in touch with nature than ever before.

For almost 30 years I've been working with both men and women in all kinds of relationships who have not been able to conceive and realise a child of their own. For many this journey is painful, frustrating and deeply saddening, but worst of all, it often gives people a great sense of injustice, as though they've been shut out of a "normal" life – excluded from the great plan of procreation – through no apparent fault of their own. Such a profound sense of hopelessness touches a deep and dark part of us, and reminds us of the pain of feeling separate from others and different.

Everyone has a unique experience. I've worked with people who have damaged fallopian tubes or low sperm counts, and with people who struggled with long-term physical health problems that they thought were unrelated to their infertility. Often there's something emotional or psychological that is getting in the way.

My husband and I had a vision of having kids and a family and we assumed it would happen the natural, easy way, and when it didn't it was a big shock. It was hard for me to get my head round it

and work out what we could do next. It's hard on your relationship because you have to re-evaluate almost every aspect of what you are together.
JOANNE

The UK has a "Fertility Industry" worth more than £600m a year, with one in six couples facing fertility problems in some form. There are 85 licensed medical clinics in the UK offering services such as in-vitro fertilisation (IVF), intra-cytoplasmic sperm injection (ICSI), egg donation, sperm donation and even treatments to suppress a woman's immune system in case it's attacking newly implanted embryos. You can take special fertility supplements made of high-dose vitamins or algae, or stock up with homeopathic remedies and follow a diet calculated to maximise your baby-making potential. There are travel companies offering "fertility retreats" where couples have massages and do yoga and qi gong.

Once a year at Olympia in London you can attend the Fertility Show where many of the clinics and practitioners specialising in fertility have stands and give out leaflets. You see bedraggled, dazzled-looking couples wandering around with handfuls of leaflets, trying to get their heads round competing packages of treatments and counselling and pampering. You can even have a fertility horoscope drawn up to calculate the right time to have sex and conceive.

Meanwhile the headlines bring new scare stories every day: "Sperm counts falling!", "Are women leaving it too late to have a baby?", "IVF babies born with fertility problems!", "Are you secretly infertile and don't know it?", "Infertility epidemic sweeps the Western world!". Friends suggest old wives-tales' – standing on your head after sex or eating kiwi fruit "because it's good for fertility" – and your mum mutters that they didn't have these problems in her day and a colleague at work unhelpfully says she only has to look at her husband to get pregnant.

The awful thing about infertility is you feel very unfeminine when everyone else is getting pregnant and you can't. It makes you feel like a complete failure as a woman. You feel very guilty that you're doing something bad and that's why it's not working. You think if only I'd had that vitamin or if I hadn't had that stressful phone conversation half an hour before the treatment. You become paranoid about everything that you do. ELIZABETH

It can be the hardest thing in the world when people turn round and say, "Look at your daughter – she's so beautiful and you're so blessed to have her," while they're surrounded by their three children, and you almost want to ask them how they'd react if one of their children were taken away from them. Secondary infertility is hard because you know what you're missing. These little beings are such cherubs. It can be difficult to realise that you won't do what you always thought you would, and have more, so you will literally do anything to change that. VALERIE

In the middle of this onslaught of advice and advertising and recommendations and counter-recommendations, it's hard to know how to stand back and calmly decide what you want to do when you are having difficulty conceiving, especially when your emotions are running high. What should be the simplest thing in the world has suddenly become a maze of options.

People with infertility issues often find themselves on a conveyor belt of treatment: first, when trying to conceive naturally fails, they are tested and diagnosed, then they are put on drugs to enhance ovulation. Then there's intra-uterine insemination (IUI), to give nature another helping hand, and if and when that fails, IVF and then ICSI, when a single sperm is injected directly into a waiting egg in a petri dish, and the resulting embryo returned to the mother for implantation.

If several cycles fail, one can look into egg or sperm donation – an option complicated by a shortage of donors and difficulties with implantation – or begin, belatedly and in a demoralised state, the long path to adopting a child.

Over the years I've worked with a huge number of patients who have had children after reaching one stage or the next of this conveyor belt and, while I think there's nothing wrong with offering medical help to couples who have difficulty conceiving, sometimes this kind of intervention wasn't needed in the first place. The achievements of modern medicine can be little short of miraculous (and many of the people I see come for acupuncture while they go through a process like IVF or ICSI or the implantation of a donor egg), but I do believe that many of these clinics don't take into account the whole person, at great cost.

The majority have a very linear, logical approach, which deals only with the basic mechanics of introducing gamete to gamete and hoping that they "take" and it can leave the newly dubbed "patients" feeling dispirited and hollow. They've been sidelined as a couple, and they're "sick" or "faulty" and mysteriously "wrong" when they'd thought they felt well in themselves only a few months before.

In 2010 the Human Fertilisation and Embryology Authority reported that only 32.2 per cent of IVF cycles performed on women under the age of 35 ended in the birth of a baby. For older women, the success rate was still worse. There is a great deal of mystery around the low success rate of IVF, even when healthy embryos are created for implantation. It's understandable that we're so concerned about infertility being epidemic, and that medical treatment isn't a guaranteed solution.

Around ten per cent of all people who visit fertility clinics are told they are simply infertile and ten per cent come away with an "unexplained infertility" diagnosis – meaning every test has been run and no physical reason can be found for the couples' failure to conceive: the woman is ovulating, the man producing sperm, everything seems to be set up and ready to go, and yet there's no child.

It's a doctor's job to give a definitive answer to this conundrum, so unexplained infertility is an unsatisfactory diagnosis for them, leaving nothing to pinpoint and calibrate and finally "cure". To the patient it's a sword of Damocles. Nothing apparently is wrong with their bodies, but something is wrong with *them* and nobody can tell them what it is. There are plenty of suggestions: not enough salmon in your diet, too much salmon, shorts too tight, ovaries just need a boost. The search for a reason can be an endless parade of possibilities, and for those involved it feels like a tremendously personal diagnosis, leaving no one to blame but yourself.

It is also regularly reported that a large percentage of "older" women, those over the age of 35, go through fertility problems. A tiny percentage of those women have passed through the menopause, but for the rest there is no explanation other than the controversial "ageing eggs" one as to why conception should be so difficult.

Let's face it, getting pregnant should be easy. People get pregnant without meaning to all the time. Two healthy human beings of childbearing years come together and have sex and, given the right timing and conditions, the egg and the sperm meet and new life begins. Mother Nature makes the babies and does everything in her power to perform her art, unless something or someone gets in her way.

Maybe it's how we're living our lives, or what we are eating, or how we are feeling each day; maybe it's just bad luck, but from my experience a failure to conceive is normally something we can change – so we need to pay close attention if we want to be in the optimum state to work with nature and increase our chances of having a child.

Nature teaches us that a balanced state is a fertile state; and in this book I would like to share with you how "balance" can be the secret to successful conception, even when all else has failed. I will help you recognise if you are in balance, and if you're not, suggest ways to achieve it.

This word "balance" is loosely defined as a state of equilibrium and we are familiar with its usage in expressions like "work/life balance", "a balanced diet", "a balanced mind", and so on. However it is easy to overlook the subtlety of this natural phenomenon and forget that everything in life must be balanced in order to function well. For example, each day is balanced by night, winter is balanced by summer, men balance women, and one of the outcomes of this particular pairing is the creation of new life – a baby.

Unexplained Infertility

In my experience, the cause of "unexplained infertility" is rarely just a physical, medical condition but more often than not something emotional or even spiritual. In the Western world we've created a society that often undermines us as unique individuals and distances us from who we truly are. We struggle in a way that previous generations did not, and even though we live in a world of relative peace and prosperity where our chances should be better than ever, they are not. The more our lives become "spiritually" unbalanced the less likely the problem of infertility will go away.

A lot of people react negatively when they hear the word "spiritual". They think you're talking about religious faith, or something mystical, but the meaning of "spirit" as understood in the philosophy that underpins Five-Element acupuncture and many other ancient healing traditions is something very different. In these systems of medicine, good health is achieved by maintaining a balance of body, mind and spirit. "Body" is our actual physical form. "Mind" is a little less tangible. Our "mind" creates our perceived reality through thought and feelings and constructs our life through experience and memories and is responsible for processing ideas. But, while everyone understands the "body" and "mind" of that equation, they tend to shy away from the third. "Spirit" is our "being" or "self", intangible and beyond thought, form, time and a sense of our own existence; "spirit" is the root and balancing point of everything.

If you and your partner are having trouble conceiving and there is no apparent medical cause then you are likely to feel deeply confused, that surely there must be something at play? To compare yourself with others who have conceived in what appears to be a similar situation to your own is frankly pointless and disheartening. We are all different: our genetic history, our personal history, our friendships, our hopes and fears.

In this book I will explain how the balance of your body, mind and spirit is crucial to your fertility. Our being will give its best when all the elements of existence are present and in equilibrium. Yes, some people are able to conceive despite having problems, but if you have had a verdict of "unexplained infertility" or there are other diagnoses that make conception harder for you, then you can increase your chances by taking a fresh look at yourself and doing everything you can to be as well as is humanly possible. When we talk about making babies we are talking about a very natural process. When we tap into the abundance of nature, which celebrates itself by reproducing, we need to be in a position to make optimum use of it.

"Unexplained infertility" to my mind is nothing more than a label and not a state of being into which you've sunk, nor is it a chronic or intractable condition. This label, however, serves as an alarm bell that tells us something is wrong and more often than not the answers are there to be found – if only we knew where to look. This is what I want to talk about in this book. It's not your average fertility guide. It asks some big questions and brings up some big concepts.

Many excellent guides to conception and conventional fertility treatments are available which will give you a detailed account of what to expect when you embark on using one treatment or another, and which will help you make informed choices. What I hope to do in this book is offer another perspective that can help you achieve a successful outcome and greatly improve your life as a whole. It takes a philosophical rather than a prescriptive approach and, hopefully, serves as a fertility-enhancing experience in itself.

Many of the people I see need medical intervention to have children, and I have nothing against the use of this when there is a clear diagnosis that supports the chosen treatment. I just advocate a balanced perspective. Hormonal treatments can be physically and emotionally gruelling, and you have to remain both optimistic and aware of the odds of success. I am concerned at times with the way that the mainstream fertility industry works, particularly the way that many patients are encouraged to seek assisted fertility far too early, to my mind, and how patients can be abruptly treated or dismissed by some clinics and consultants. In spite of these concerns, I have witnessed amazing results thanks to medical treatment.

My primary intention, either when working with individuals one on one or by sharing with you in this book, is to help awaken and discover the truth of who you really are. As you begin to recognise and break old habits, and dispel myths and unhelpful ideas that burden your mind, you will start to make choices that speak best to your true sense of self. This heightened awareness and clarity bring health to all aspects of your life. By being authentic, you will find a renewed sense of balance that will realign you with everything in your life.

There are no buttons that will simply switch fertility on or off. The relationships between the human body, mind and spirit are as complex as nature itself. My job and the job of everyone in the fertility industry, be they a doctor, psychotherapist or acupuncturist, is to help move the person to a balanced place where the natural force of creation can dominate, resulting in a successful pregnancy. The energy that creates and sees life thrive is available to all of us. We just need to provide the right conditions within ourselves to allow this life force to circulate and nourish us.

Every day in my work I see people improving in their physical and mental health, changing their lives for the better and often falling pregnant in spite of an earlier diagnosis of "unexplained infertility". However, I am not blind in my optimism; I'm a pragmatist. It's not enough to simply turn up and receive this or that treatment. A certain focus, rigour and determination are needed to become a "healthy instrument" – but, believe me, the potential for a life-changing shift *is* there in you, whether it results in you having longed-for children, or just living a better, happier life.

Throughout this book I will use stories from people I have helped which I hope will show that infertility isn't a simple issue, but one that requires a holistic approach – i.e. one that takes you and many aspects of your life into account. People come to professionals like me with many different problems and leave with many different solutions. Some of the case studies are brief, and others more detailed, provided from the perspective of the people themselves. All of these stories reach a conclusion, and the outcomes are often surprising. I hope they will guide you to find your own path through the choices before you, and to emerge at the other end of your journey feeling more at peace and better in your own skin.

I will use these stories to highlight how certain beliefs and ways of thinking can be counterproductive to your fertility; how to recognise these negative thought patterns in yourself, and how to make positive change.

I will also explain the Five-Element philosophy which underpins the acupuncture treatment that many of these people received. This explanation will show how the ancient wisdom contained in this system of medicine can be hugely beneficial to you, even without the insertion of a needle. While the philosophy behind the Five Elements may seem alien at first, I hope to demonstrate how it underlies even our Western, 21st-century lives.

A Holistic Approach

Jeanie and Nick Gordon had been together for seven years before they married in 2000, and twelve months later they began trying for a baby. Jeanie was 31 and Nick 34. Both of them had good jobs that they loved in London and they had been able to buy their own flat. It seemed like the perfect set-up for starting a family and everything had gone according to plan, but two years on there had been no positive pregnancy tests, and the couple found themselves surrounded by friends who were producing babies and even second babies without any problems.

Their GP referred them to a specialist who examined and tested both of them and found that Nick's sperm were not very active, and that Jeanie hadn't ovulated on her last cycle. A scan revealed that Jeanie had a large fibroid, which had twisted one of her fallopian tubes back on itself. An operation to remove it worked, and after a month off work to recover, Jeanie felt refreshed and hopeful about the chances of becoming pregnant. She carried on with her timetabled visits to the gym and the vitamin supplements she'd been recommended, cutting back on alcohol just to be careful. Nick drank rather more and smoked a packet of cigarettes each day, but both the couple's GP and their consultant assured them that it would probably be stressful and therefore harmful for Nick, a committed smoker, to quit the habit.

Six months later, the couple had not conceived and Jeanie was under increasing stress. A friend who already had a child had just tested pregnant with twins. Although Jeanie had never experienced bad PMT, she now began to go through an enormous emotional and physical crash each month when her period began, and end up sobbing under her duvet or drinking too much and being so hung-over the next day that she had to phone in sick. Nick was hugely supportive all this time, but the couple were advised by their GP to move on to

IVF. Jeanie had just changed jobs from a place where she'd had difficulties, and hoped that this would remove some of the stress.

Jeanie started taking large doses of the drug Clomid – that stimulates the pituitary gland to promote ovulation – so that some of her eggs could be gathered and fertilised with Nick's sperm. The side effects of the drugs were grim – constant abdominal pain and mood swings – but the couple were determined to see it through. They were using ICSI which differs from conventional IVF in that the embryologist selects a single sperm to be injected directly into an egg, instead of placing lots of sperm in a dish with one egg – so only a few quality sperm would be needed and all Nick had to do was produce a sample. Although she felt under huge pressure, Jeanie reacted well to the treatment and produced a good quantity of eggs, most of which were frozen after fertilisation for future rounds of ICSI.

They were overjoyed when Jeanie tested pregnant after their first attempt. However, an early scan indicated problems with the foetus, and at eight and a half weeks Jeanie miscarried while staying at her sister's house. As her sister had just announced that she'd got pregnant after only three months of trying, Jeanie concealed what had happened from her, even driving herself to hospital with crippling stomach cramps. She later said that it felt like all her hope had gone with the pregnancy. Although her boss was understanding, going back to work was difficult as the new job wasn't working out.

Half a year later they tried a second round of ICSI, and this time when Jeanie conceived she carried on using hormone patches to help the pregnancy. Six weeks in, the scan showed that the foetus had been lost and Jeanie broke down in the car as they drove home. They had had enough. Jeanie was exhausted and exasperated at bearing the burden of the treatments, and was beginning to feel that her body had let her down. They both knew that something had to change.

Jeanie had been looking at fertility treatments in acupuncture, reflexology and Chinese herbs. When a friend recommended our clinic, she decided to book an appointment for herself and Nick. At this stage, they hoped that acupuncture would help support further ICSI procedures and give the embryo a better chance of implanting. I saw the couple jointly for an initial consultation, and then separately for their actual treatment. Jeanie describes her experiences:

Some of the tips given to us seemed very practical and straightforward – things like drinking more water and less coffee; but Gerad also tackled Nick on the question of his health and the link with his low-sperm motility. Nick never ate breakfast or lunch, in fact he often didn't eat till ten o'clock at night, and he was dreadful at getting out of bed in the morning. At the weekends he'd sleep in till two in the afternoon. Gerad's advice to him was to eat either scrambled eggs and smoked salmon or a bacon sandwich for breakfast every morning, which of course Nick thought was fantastic. I thought it was fantastic too as over the weeks, I saw his energy levels changing. He was less sluggish in the mornings, and got up earlier at weekends.

To me it was a huge relief that he wasn't let off the hook any more. With the fertility treatments we'd had earlier, all he'd had to do was provide a couple of samples, but now for the first time it really felt like we were in it together. I poured my heart out, and it was so nice to sit down with somebody and let off steam – you didn't feel like you were out in the cold any more. It also felt like it was the whole of me that was being treated, and not just the baby-making bits.

During the first treatment I remember having needles put in points down my back and left in for a while, and it felt like someone was pouring a jug of cold water over my back. It was a really weird sensation. Afterwards I felt positively trippy. It was like being on holiday, when you've forgotten to worry about everything and things look different; instead of saying "Oh God, look at the traffic", you're all "Oh! Cars! How lovely!" I asked him to tone it down a bit the next time! I began to get the sense that it would all work out OK.

After a couple of sessions we went away on holiday and that was when I decided to give up work. I don't think I'd have had the courage to walk out if it hadn't been for the acupuncture. I was a bit disappointed that I didn't turn out to be pregnant on that cycle, but I didn't go through a huge hormonal crash like the ones I'd experienced before. I did my final day at work a month later and two days after that we discovered that I was pregnant. In June 2006 our son Tom was born.

Jeanie and Nick's case is a perfect illustration of the kind of story and outcome we have seen with many of our patients. Jeanie clearly needed medical help to diagnose and remove the fibroid that was affecting her chances of conceiving, and yet the consultants whom the couple visited apparently saw nothing wrong with Nick's lifestyle, and didn't believe it could be affecting the quality of his sperm and their chances of conceiving. Acupuncture helped Jeanie to let go of much of the stress and anger she'd gone through while trying to conceive, and she was relieved to leave a stressful and unpleasant workplace. Nick made practical changes to his life which ended up having a huge impact. In the end they didn't need to use IVF or ICSI to have their child.

Many patients attribute their improvement to the balancing nature of acupuncture treatment alone, but often their breakthrough involves a combination of help from hypnotherapy, counselling, IVF, surgery and even, like Nick and Jeanie, changing jobs or making other lifestyle changes. Nothing is a definite cure and a complex problem can require many solutions. I hope that reading about their experience and the other stories in this book will help you to take an open-minded approach to that maze of options, and to see that even the smallest shift in attention can affect necessary change.

An Accidental Expert

When I started to practise Five-Element acupuncture I had no intention of specialising in infertility. My reputation as a "fertility expert" took off after I helped a single patient who wanted a cure for hay fever and got more than she bargained for.

At the time I was working for the NHS at Kings College Hospital part-time, mainly treating patients with HIV/Aids and other immune-related disorders, and I'd set up a private practice in south London treating all kinds of symptoms including allergies, back pain and helping people quit smoking.

One of my first private patients, Maggie, was 40,

married, worked as a solicitor and had one son, aged ten. After the first treatment she was delighted; her hay fever symptoms had disappeared completely and she was feeling surprisingly relaxed and just like her old self. I was delighted to get such a swift result too, and Maggie immediately referred three of her friends to my practice.

A month later Maggie made a new appointment, but this time she seemed even less well than when I'd first met her. She wasn't very impressed by me. It was June and her hay fever had recurred, leaving her feeling exhausted and irritable. I tentatively gave her a second treatment, hoping it would do the trick this time. When she returned for a third session she was a different woman again: still exhausted, but she was absolutely ecstatic and could barely wait till she was in the treatment room to tell me her news: she was pregnant! She hadn't told me during her first consultation that she'd been trying to get pregnant for a second time for years and had been diagnosed as having "secondary infertility" five years previously.

Within weeks two of Maggie's friends whom she had referred bounced into the treatment room with the same fanfare, also surprising me – neither of them had mentioned that they were trying to conceive, and I'd thought they'd come to me for stress-related problems. This flurry of surprise pregnancies caused a minor stir in south London and suddenly I was besieged by women who wanted the same magical instant-conception treatment. I found myself having to explain that I wasn't treating infertility per se – rather, my treatments were aimed at helping nature restore balance.

Let me explain the underlying philosophy of the treatments given, as the teachings are useful in helping you understand the importance of "balance" to your fertility.

The Nature of Balance

Five-Element acupuncture evolved in China more than 5000 years ago as a comprehensive system of medicine. This ancient culture had a profound understanding of the connection between the laws of nature and good health. And acupuncture treatment was designed to balance the patient's system so that it functioned optimally, which in turn eradicated disease and improved the quality of the patient's overall health. When the women in south London who came to me for treatment fell pregnant it really was an accident, or, more accurately, a side effect of a bigger change that had taken place in them.

The notion of not treating something in order to treat it is very Chinese. Whereas we in the West want things to make linear sense, the Chinese love contradictions and so an understanding of ancient Chinese "thought" is helpful in making the connection between, say, hay fever and irritable bowel syndrome or depression and infertility.

In the West it is normal to wait until we're sick before we seek help. Preventative medicine is seen as alternative and rather unsatisfying because it fails to meet our results-orientated society. Our medical system is more focused on curing cancer than preventing it in the first place. No one talks about the person who doesn't get sick, but we all love a story of someone overcoming a potentially fatal disease and the cast of heroes who swoop in to save the day. Surgeons in our culture are like gods. In ancient China they were seen as butchers who stepped in when the physician had failed.

"Treating the person", a common expression in Five-Element acupuncture, means making sure the body, mind and spirit of the person are functioning in a balanced and harmonious way. When everything is in order, symptoms will go away and we are well and can thrive.

A good analogy is that of a house and how it provides the right environment for the family who lives there to be happy and healthy. The walls, windows and roof need to be well maintained and secure, the plumbing must carry fresh water throughout the house, the drains must carry away the waste. The boiler heats the water for radiators and the rooms ought to be decorated in a pleasant and stimulating way. By creating an environment that meets the needs of the family, it is more likely that within it there will be a balanced and pleasant existence free from sickness and pain. All of the factors involved – the heat, the water, the structure, the removal of waste, the décor – are interconnected, and if one is knocked out of sync the whole is affected. If the roof leaks, the walls will rot, the heating system will go on pumping out warm air that is lost to a draught and soon everyone in the house is sick.

I see a lot of people whose metaphorical houses are falling down around their ears, but who will swear blind that everything would be just fine if only they could sort out their wheat intolerance or stop having hay fever or start having babies. The majority of those patients who come for treatment for infertility believe that acupuncture will strengthen their reproductive system and help it to perform. To some extent that's true, but what the treatment really does is reconnect the patient with something much more powerful than any conventional treatment or medication – their own innate intelligence and ability to find balance and return to optimum health.

The reason most of us seek help from a professional is that we have lost the ability to maintain balance and self-heal. And we trust that it is often much easier for a third party to see what's going on with us, since, by the time we reach our thirties and forties, we've been adjusting to minor symptoms and negative ways of being for so long that we find our physiological ebb and flow all completely normal. This is particularly true of patients diagnosed with "unexplained infertility" who have no obvious fertility-related symptoms but more often than not many other minor problems.

The Five-Element practitioner has very particular skills to diagnose and treat imbalances, and can even detect a potential problem before any symptoms show. For example, if you came to me as a new patient and told me you had headaches, irregular periods and mild depression, I'd have to confess that your symptoms simply tell me you're out of balance and little else. The symptoms themselves don't say anything to me about how to treat you in the first instance, as they are just alarm bells saying there is something wrong, and it certainly would not be responsible of me to try to turn off the alarm bell before I've found the cause. Rather than try and do something directly about those nagging superficial symptoms, my job is to head straight to the root of the problem.

The role of the Five-Element practitioner is to care for the patient in the widest sense, to listen, to understand, to develop an authentic relationship, and then to interpret the entire experience through an intelligent and effective treatment that addresses the cause and will restore balance and help the person out of suffering.

The signs and signals we look for are not necessarily those that a Western doctor would use for diagnosis, and as I said we do not treat symptoms directly when we find them. Where a doctor might provide an anti-histamine to stop a patient's eyes feeling itchy and their nose running from hay fever, a Five-Element acupuncturist wants to uncover the true cause of why a person's system is out of balance and thus made them more vulnerable to illness.

"Traditional Chinese Medicine" or "TCM" is the most widespread type of acupuncture that you are likely to find in your town centre or on your high street, and it differs from Five-Element acupuncture. When Chairman Mao, the Communist leader, came to power in 1949, he needed a rudimentary health service to serve the growing Chinese population and get them back to work if they fell sick. This new regime shut down many educational institutions and drove practitioners of all styles of acupuncture out of work – the spiritual aspect of their type of medicine being regarded as elitist, superstitious and outdated. The Chinese people reacted strongly to this change, however, demanding that acupuncture be reinstated, so Mao ordered the creation of a new style of acupuncture, which was modernised, standardised and rolled out across the nation. It was a system that laid out recommended formulas and acupuncture points to use for treating this or that specific syndrome or physical disorder. These new state acupuncturists kept the same body map of points and the skills of pulse-taking previously used, but the core spiritual Taoist philosophy behind the treatment was greatly reduced and the whole practice reformulated. TCM, like Western medicine, focuses primarily on the presenting symptoms and aims to eradicate those, and while it is highly effective, it's similar to palliative care.

Many of the current studies into how acupuncture aids fertility look specifically at the treatment of organs and functions that directly relate to conception. This is then measured to evaluate the number of conceptions that result. For a Five-Element practitioner, this results-led approach is all wrong: our focus is not just on fertility and the intention is not to "make" couples conceive – in fact, we can't; the best we can do is help a patient's system find its way back to balance and thereby let their internal mechanism do the work.

The body, mind and spirit naturally seek balance, and the acupuncturist just facilitates this. For example, in a patient presenting with, let's say, backache, along with a lack of confidence and infertility, these individual symptoms are not targeted one by one, but treated simultaneously as internal homeostasis is restored. I can say that a treatment has been truly successful only if the patient ends the process feeling thoroughly well in body, mind and spirit, with their symptoms addressed and energy restored. That happy state may or may not include a baby.

A Philosophical Approach

So what is this ancient Chinese philosophy, and how is it useful to you?

"Taoist" philosophy sees the universe in paired terms: night and day, black and white, male and female. The ancient Chinese believed that heaven represented the father, earth represented the mother, and they, the humans, were the offspring of nature, created and maintained by these two parents. Everything we see around us is the creation of the two primary forces of the mother and the father. You're probably familiar with the black and white symbol of yin and yang. Taoists see heaven as yang – fatherly, lighter and predominantly non-material; and earth as yin – motherly, darker and predominantly material.

We humans live and experience everything between these two poles and we are sustained throughout our lives by each heavenly breath we inspire from our "father", and every earthly morsel of food we ingest from our "mother". We're a combination of material and non-material, and our challenge is to balance the two, and if we're successful we will, in theory, thrive, reproduce and survive for a hundred years! When we fail to maintain that balance, we get sick, and as long as we are sick our symptoms remind us we've lost that balance.

The dynamic coming together and reaction of the

two poles of material and non-material, heaven and earth, perfection and imperfection, also produces the Five Elements: wood, fire, earth, metal and water: our world. Everything in existence is made up of a compound of these elements found in nature, and human beings are no exception. We exist as all five, and the balance of those elements is unique to each of us, and can also vary by the day or even the hour. To return to my earlier analogy, the elements are the impermanent components of the house – the heating, the walls, the roof, and so on – they are what make us unique, and make up our personality. They are in a constant state of change. The permanent "self" at our core is the origin or foundation of the house. That "self" is who we really are and is constant - our whole potential and the Five Elements enable that potential to come to fruition, as an outer, projected impermanent, or temporary, structure – the house.

Each of the Five Elements has certain qualities and associations that can be related to every aspect of the human experience. They shape our physical bodies, internal organs and systems, organise our thoughts and fuel our feelings and give our life form; they also make babies.

For you to be in the fullness of who you are as a human being, and have the capacity to express yourself and reproduce, all Five Elements need to be present, engaged and working together to maintain a balanced relationship with one another. In this healthy state, all the elements maintain equilibrium, adjusting for each new situation life presents and then settling back into place, or reconfiguring ready to tackle each fresh challenge. When you respond to situations spontaneously and appropriately, you can roll with the constant flux of life. Making a baby is no different; each of the Five Elements has an assigned role and responds to the intricate process of creating new life. A natural homeostasis operates in everything, a universal life force working in us all to guide us through the turbulence of the human experience and back to a harmonious state, which survives us when we die.

However, part of the challenge of being a human is that each person has a flaw, a kind of Achilles heel or imbalance rooted in one of the Five Elements. It's a default setting that we all have, consistent with the dualistic nature of life, and is the original cause of all imbalances in us.

Professor JR Worsley, who was one of my teachers and credited with bringing Five-Element acupuncture to the West, believed and taught that every human being has one original elemental imbalance, or "causative factor", that remains constant throughout his or her life regardless of the current state of health. We can easily slip with the pressures of life, and any or all of the elements can suffer as a result. However, this slip will always be rooted in the person's weakest element, and all problems, mental, physical and spiritual, stem from this place. This is a significant starting point when looking for the causes of unexplained infertility. And, for any Five-Element acupuncturist of Worsley's tradition, identifying that element is essential to treating a patient successfully. It is the key to getting that person back on track. For our purposes, however, an understanding of each of the elements and how they function in you will provide you with an awareness of whether you are in balance, and more importantly, how you are not. When you gain greater insight into how you function and behave, any necessary change becomes an immediate possibility, in turn positively affecting your general health and your fertility.

Finding Balance

So how do we know if one, or all of the elements, are imbalanced in us?

The moment any one of the Five Elements becomes distressed it immediately sends out a signal asking for help, and this will be apparent in many different ways. A Five-Element acupuncturist looks for and diagnoses a patient's "causative factor" – the primary elemental imbalance – by paying attention to a colour that shows on the face around their eyes, a sound in their voice, an odour and a predominant emotion. For example, in a patient with a "causative factor" in the earth element, the colour will be yellow, their voice will have a sing-song sound, they will smell slightly sweet and crave understanding and sympathy. In a patient with a "causative factor" in the wood element, the colour will be green, their voice will have a clipped sound, the smell will be "rancid" and they will appear frustrated and angry. As human faces, voices, odours and emotions come in every variation, this might seem a rather curious statement to make – how could the whole of mankind possibly appear in just five ways that relate to a distress call in one of the Five Elements?

The answer is that these distress signals underlie all other factors, because it's nature's way of alerting us to the cause of the problem. To the very skilled diagnostician, it is obvious. And, actually, although it can take years to develop an expertise in recognising these signs in others, we do *all* have this instinctual ability, whether we are acupuncturists or not. The more we awaken from our slumber and pay attention to what nature is telling us, the more obvious this kind of information becomes.

We react all the time to smells in the street even if only unconsciously, crossing the road without thinking, or suddenly feeling hungry because of a whiff of fresh bread from a bakery. We know when someone in front of us in a queue is agitated or threatening. Think of the way that a mother can catch a tone in her child's voice before more than a dozen words are said on the phone and know instantly that he or she is sad, excited, angry or in need. Parents watch their children, their lovers and partners the whole time. If we pick up the slightest change in their complexions and smells, we react. It doesn't matter what they say, because we have already sensed the direction their feelings have taken. I've often reflected that, if you took away our senses and left us with only words, no one would have a clue what was going on.

It's always very exciting when I walk into a room with a new patient waiting as there will be one predominant odour in the room that is being produced by one of the elements that will speak to me to help me make a diagnosis, and is nothing to do with sweat, perfume or unwashed clothes. To the expert nose, someone who is very imbalanced can give off an element odour so strong that it's quite disconcerting at first.

For the layperson, registering someone's emotional or physical state is not so conscious, but still at some primitive, instinctive level we are at it all the time and we certainly use these natural skills for our own survival. Becoming conscious and being able to read coded information about our self and others is particularly useful at a time of sickness and confusion. Understanding what nature is telling us not only provides the answers to what we are looking for, but brings a sense of calm, with our tolerance and compassion for ourselves and others enhanced.

As I go on with the explanation of Taoist Five-Element philosophy, you will see that the Chinese recognised that everything in life is interconnected, and that when one part of the whole is affected, this will in turn affect everything else, as in the description of the house in the first chapter.

The Five Elements correspond to five Chinese seasons: wood in spring, fire in summer, earth in late summer, metal in autumn and water in winter. Each season, like each element, is a manifestation of nature as it goes through its cycle – growth in spring, flowering in summer, harvest in late summer, decomposition in autumn and regeneration in winter: five stages of one year.

The elements are also responsible for the creation and maintenance of the organs, parts and functions of the human body, because we are part of nature and our physical structure mirrors that of our external world. This microcosm of the human body is scaled up to nature as a whole, like a larger but otherwise identical Russian doll. For example, in the same way that the convection cycle draws water from rivers, lakes and oceans to form clouds which descend on mountains and come back down to earth as nourishing rain, so our kidneys and bladder control the water in our body, cleansing, lubricating and providing enormous reserves of flowing energy.

Chinese medicine differs greatly from Western medicine in the way it sees the purpose and role of our internal organs and functions. In the Chinese system the organs and functions, also known as "Officials", have specific responsibilities that deal with not only the physical, but every other aspect of being human. Taking the previous example of the kidneys and bladder, not only do these two "Officials" process fluids, they also govern our drive and ambition, our ability to find stillness and peace, and our instinct to survive – to name but a few. Unlike the Western approach of compartmentalising organ functions and diseases, the Chinese system sees the complex internal relationships of our organs and functions extending to every aspect of our overall health. It's essential to grasp this interconnectedness when looking at the possible causes of infertility and what is required to conceive. As well as air, water and food, we take in vast quantities of information and life experience from the outside world that affect us both positively and negatively, and the organs and functions each have a role in processing those influxes.

Most infertility treatments, both conventional and alternative, tend to concentrate on the reproductive organs and the endocrine system that governs our hormones, without considering the other organs and systems which underpin, supply and support them. But, as we shall see, each and every one of the Five Elements is essential for creating the right conditions for successful conception and pregnancy – for example: wood for regulation of the menstrual cycle, the male erection and the growth of the foetus; fire for passion and sexual activity, temperature regulation, the warming of the womb and cooling of the testicles; earth to nourish the blood, build the uterine lining and feed the developing baby; metal to provide quality air, essential trace elements and release the waste; and water for the power of creation, regulation of the hormonal flow and maturation of healthy eggs and sperm.

As you read on and learn more about the elements and their associated organs and functions, it may seem that there are some surprising omissions – the brain, for example, or the uterus – but these fall under the category of secondary or "extraordinary" organs in the Chinese system. Since this is a guide to baby-making rather than a textbook on Five-Element acupuncture, I will concentrate on the primary organs and functions directly associated with each of the elements, how they contribute to a balanced state of being and how when they are out of balance they will produce symptoms that negatively affect your fertility. I will also give a number of case studies to show how when an element is in distress it can be detrimental to the person in question on many levels.

There is no expectation or need for you to diagnose

yourself from what you read. But you will recognise bits of yourself in the elements, some more than others, and hopefully the descriptions of the elements and the characters in the case studies will help you recognise where you yourself might be out of balance and struggling, where possibly you need to make changes – and maybe even ask for help.

The Five Elements

Wood

The wood element is associated with spring. The Five-Element acupuncturist's diagnosis for a person with an imbalance in this element is the colour green showing in the face, a "rancid" odour, a shouting or tight, clipped timbre to the voice, and a primary emotion of anger, or a lack of anger. To anyone reared on the principles of Western medicine, this might seem rather strange, but Chinese medical philosophy takes a very nuanced approach, which embraces the patterns of life on multiple levels. According to their belief system, wood is associated with spring, and spring is a time when everything comes alive and begins to expand and grow. There is a sense of relief and freedom as vegetation that died or went underground in winter starts to grow again, and new animals are born. Just when most of nature seemed to be dead it is revealed to have been sleeping all along. For us this also means everything awakens and now feels possible, and so it's a time to make plans and employ strategies to move on.

Imagine, then, what happens when this natural cycle is stopped in its tracks. Imagine being a seed underground ready to burst forth and then a paving slab being placed on the ground above you, which stops your action and all your potential. How would you feel? The Chinese pictogram for "anger" is of a tree growing in a box; something that is not allowed to grow healthily in an unchecked fashion. When you have a primary imbalance in the wood element you have a feeling of being restricted, frustrated and angry: either you have an abnormal amount of anger that comes shooting out of you at the slightest provocation, or else you feel defeated, devoid of the assertiveness that could help you move and change, and yet under this seemingly passive state you feel angry, resigned and depressed. We tend to see anger as a negative emotion, and it can be when it is not used well, or when it flares up strongly, but it's also a driving force; if we do not grow and develop as nature intends, the whole cycle of life can feel as if it has ended before it has begun.

Wood is seen as holding the plan of life and provides the strategy for all action. It provides the direction and focus for what the body, mind and spirit are going to do and how they are going to keep going and survive. Because our primary job as human beings is to be who we are and bring the uniqueness and fullness of ourselves into the world, we need this element to give us vision and clarity so that we can see ourselves and our situation clearly enough to take action as our life unfolds. If something gets in our way, we need the flexibility either to engage and make change or find a way to adapt rather than simply becoming blocked and stuck.

Wood's associated organs are the gall bladder and the liver. Physiologically the gall bladder produces and secretes bile to assist in the breakdown of fats, which helps with the digestive process. Digestion continues through the digestive tract and nutrients then pass into the blood, entering the liver, which further purifies and passes these life-giving substances on to the rest of the body.

Five-Element acupuncture ascribes a further role to the gall bladder and liver – that of organising and directing all the body's other organs. Any action that materialises in life requires a plan and a decision. Our immune system can't fight off infections if it doesn't strike and attack a foreign body; the stomach cannot digest food if it doesn't have the ability to balance digestive juices, and our tendons and ligaments cannot bend and stretch without the flexibility of wood's great plan. All kinds of symptoms such as stomach ulcers, irritable bowel syndrome, menstrual cramps and irregular menstruation can result when the wood element is not functioning correctly.

The bottled-up frustration often seen with an imbalance in wood also leads to physical symptoms like tension pain from wrought-up muscles, RSI, headaches, eye problems, weak nails, poor digestion and even breathing problems.

I am often alerted to a patient with a wood imbalance as soon as I walk into the waiting room at the clinic. The first hint: although subtle, a look of suppressed anger, and then all smiles and politeness on greeting; they almost crush my hand as I shake it. Others are self-effacing to the point of timidity, but you find that if you hit the wrong subject they're primed to erupt. Patients who come for treatment are often not aware that the way they feel or behave is strange in any way – it's all they know. If you ask if they are frustrated or angry they will look surprised and vehemently deny it, or blame their mood on an external thing, or perhaps others around them whom they deem inconsiderate or annoying.

Wood: a case study

"They told me there was parking nearby – and there's not!" Ruby shot at me as we shook hands in greeting. Taken aback and confused by the soft gentle hand in mine, I pulled away, apologised for the misinformation and indicated the direction of my treatment room.

Ruby was 32, a striking-looking woman with

piercing eyes and long, floaty limbs. As she climbed the stairs in front of me I was mesmerised by her graceful flight; each movement seemed choreographed to the finest detail. Once settled in the room, she immediately opened the consultation. "I need to be pregnant by the end of June," she told me. "Otherwise I will wait until next year... Can you help me?"

She'd been with her husband for five years and had stopped taking the contraceptive pill a year before coming to me. Her periods were regular and, as she proudly told me, were running like a "Swiss clock". She was surprised and disappointed that she had not already conceived but put it down to a very erratic sex life due to both their work commitments. Her only other complaint was tension in her jaw and an ache at the back of her head. Her body was an unusual combination of super flexibility, noticeable when I lifted her arm, and absolute tension in her neck when she attempted to move her head from side to side.

As I explained how treatment works and what she could expect, I couldn't help noticing her glancing up to the ceiling and hearing her "tut-tutting" under her breath. I was clearly irritating her and anything other than the essentials of treatment seemed likely to cause her stress.

Ruby came for treatment every Tuesday morning at 8.15am. Despite being a very busy woman, she was never late. During a typical treatment, prior to inserting a needle, I warm the area over the acupuncture point with moxa, a Chinese herb that is placed and burnt over the skin. Rather than tell me when she felt the pleasant warming sensation as guided, Ruby would wait for it to burn and then scold me.

In spite of the misgivings I had at first, we worked well together and she responded to treatment. Her neck relaxed, her headaches cleared and on treatment six she arrived at 8.18am. Now I knew I was getting somewhere. Most importantly, during one session when she was lying on the treatment couch, she revealed to me that a recurrent nightmare she had had since childhood had suddenly changed. She told me the story.

When Ruby was fourteen her older brother Adam was killed in a car crash. They had been inseparable their whole lives and now without warning she was an only child. As she told me about Adam and his death she cried and gripped me so tightly she forced the blood out of my hand. Until recently, she had been dreaming that she and Adam would be walking through a field she knew and suddenly without warning he would run off with a group of his friends and be gone, no longer wanting to be seen with her.

Ruby began to relax with me as she recounted her dream, and even more so as she reported that since her acupuncture treatment had started, Adam would appear in her dream, and then stay.

Ruby conceived bang on schedule. That aspect of her

character wasn't changing, but the charge around her did, to a softer, easier, more-at-peace Ruby.

Fire

Fire is the element of summer. Unlike wood, water, earth and metal, it is associated with not only two organs – the heart and small intestine – but also two functions that don't have a physical form and are called "circulation-sex" and "three heater".

The heart was seen by the ancient Chinese as our direct connection with heaven and was considered the most important organ in the body as it pumps blood and life to every cell – a unifying action. The heart is the seat of passion and love, sending out blood unconditionally to every cell in the body to maintain life. The small intestine, known as the "separator of pure from impure", supports the heart by filtering out impurities and the detritus and irrelevance of daily life thereby leaving the heart free to receive the "mandate of heaven". The "three heater", meanwhile, maintains and regulates temperature by keeping the passageways clear and acts like a thermostat, and "circulation-sex" is, as the name suggests, responsible for the circulatory system and for our passion and sexual activity. We recognise this when we are aroused, and blood is sent to our genitals and our lips, making them fuller and more sensitive. Symbolically, the "three heater" and "circulation-sex" open our heart, our inner private self to our outer world and the hearts of others.

So what can happen when you have an imbalance in the fire element? The odour is that of burnt or scorched material. When the fire element is functioning properly, it will hold you on an even keel with an appropriate level of joy, like the comforting warmth of a farmhouse Aga. People with an imbalance in fire can "overheat", be inappropriately exuberant and demanding, and almost hysterically happy about everything. The flipped version of this is the person who cannot find joy in anything, and who withdraws from company and seems indifferent and cold. You can recognise someone with an imbalance in the fire element by the sound in their voice – it either has a relentless laughter in it, or it's sapped of emotion and flat. The colour seen on the face at each side of the patient's eyes is a reflection of that too; grey if there is too little fire, and red if there is too much.

When fire is functioning well, we unconditionally generate love for ourselves and for others and feel safe at home in our self and out in the world. We know when to open and when to close; we are at our fullest potential as individuals. However, when the fire is struggling or almost burnt out we feel vulnerable and defenceless, and lose our ability to communicate properly and openly with others, walking down the street with our eyes cast down to avoid other people's attention. People with a causative factor in fire can be quick to abandon their friends who they feel have hurt or offended them, even if to an outsider the offence doesn't seem so grave.

This inconsistency in social interaction can lead to people leaping into friendships and being desperate to be best friends straight away, at times intruding into the other person's life; there seems to be a need to almost engulf that person. They lack the subtle skill of respecting healthy boundaries and often blow hot and cold socially. Although their pathology is more apparent in emotional issues, it might also manifest itself in physical symptoms: circulation problems, heart palpitations, boils and other indicators that all is not well.

Fire: a case study

I have to confess I can't remember the name of this particular patient, as privately I affectionately called him "The Laughing Salesman". About fifteen years ago I was employed by companies to go to their offices once a week and treat some of their employees. The laughing salesman was one of my patients. I always knew when he was on his way as I could hear him whistling and chirping to himself as he came down the long echoing corridor to the treatment room. Then he'd rap on the door, fly into the room and often make a quip, or laugh. Everything he did had to be a joke. He couldn't help himself. He couldn't take anything seriously. The banter was relentless, and after a while I began to find it slightly perturbing.

He was clearly extremely good at his job as a salesman. He had boundless energy. He'd come in at 5am, drink buckets of coffee and challenge all the younger guys to a squash match in the company gym. The office was large enough for him to bounce from desk to desk telling his jokes without exasperating too many people, but you couldn't have contained him in a smaller set-up – he would have driven everyone mad.

It was another story for his wife, of course, who, it sounded to me, was exhausted with the effort of keeping up with him. Once he cheerily told me that she'd asked him to book a holiday at a nice hotel by the sea, and he'd decided that that couldn't possibly be what she wanted – far too boring – and had hired a camper van for them to drive around America instead.

The laughing salesman was only in his mid-thirties but his face was scarlet. His blood pressure was soaring and his body was permanently hot. Sometimes, it seemed to me that he'd never matured properly; it was as if he was just cooking the whole time and was never done. Some weeks into his treatment it also transpired that he had a low sperm count, and he and his wife were having difficulty conceiving.

Working with him was an uphill struggle for me and

it took a very long time to see palpable results. It was a challenge to get him to just feel neutral about something. In our culture we place a high value on joy and being "up" and try to avoid feelings that are negative or low, but too much of any emotion is bad – everything must be given its balanced expression.

Gradually, notch by notch, he lowered his defences and seemed to quieten. His high colouring began to fade and I no longer felt like I was touching a hot plate when I checked his pulse. I tried to encourage him to do something he liked, like swimming, rather than thrash around the squash court. He went from an almost total lack of self-awareness to being able to have meaningful conversations. After many months of treatment and lifestyle changes, he reported that his wife had conceived and he was going to be a dad.

Earth

The Chinese separate summer into two parts, and earth is the element connected to the harvest season of late summer when the crops are gathered and brought into granaries for winter storage. Metaphorically, you can see its connection with the associated organs; the stomach, which also takes in food and resources, and the spleen, which turns that food into energy and nourishment and stores the extra as fat for future needs.

Of the "Officials", the spleen is considered the Minister for Transport, moving everything along we take in – from ideas, to food, to all of our emotions.

The colour associated with earth is yellow, the smell is sweet, an oaty one of fermentation, and the sound in the voice is a sing-song, a bit like a lullaby, as when a mother speaks to her child. People with a causative factor in earth seem to be primarily caught up in nurturing and sympathy (or the lack thereof). This element is responsible for the way we care or look after ourselves and others around us, and monitors our nourishment on all levels. Have our guests got enough to eat? Are there good books to read on the shelf? Are we all going to have the most comfortable seats on the flight? It's a kind of circular relationship of giving things out and taking them in, of interaction with our environment.

Some people whose earth element is in trouble are curled inward and stuck in their own world of feeling sorry for themselves. They believe they don't have enough. They ask for sympathy but reject it when they receive it. It's as though they think they have no choice but to function without any true interaction with others, while at the same time it's obvious to a bystander that they need help.

Equally, the reverse can be true. People desperate to provide an environment that they believe will make you happy, and by default please them, hurl themselves into an "earth mother" role by doling out provisions, understanding and sympathy in a way that is more likely to swamp you rather than help you. If you have a headache they know exactly how it feels because they had one, only it was worse. You might just be chatting and telling them about your recent trip to the shops where you forgot your money but the intensity of their attention to your story and the resulting sympathy seem inappropriate. They have no guard or brake when it comes to giving "care".

Physically, the knock-on effect of an imbalance in this element is often seen in digestive and metabolic problems. A person seems ravenous and constantly eats but never gains weight because they can't process food properly, or else they don't know when to stop as no matter how much they eat they never feel satisfied. Feeling this emptiness, they keep on eating and of course their body packs on fat. They are often groggy physically and mentally because, although they are continually taking everything on board, very little is getting processed and sent to the right place. Other symptoms include gastric reflux, bloating and flatulence – even recurrent miscarriage. When earth is balanced, however, a person knows exactly how much food to eat or information to process or emotion to absorb, and certainly when to stop.

Earth: a case study

When I think of an example of somebody with an imbalance in the earth element, my lovely patient Sarah springs to mind. She was in her late thirties when she came to see me for help. She'd been involved with a married man, 20 years older than her for nearly two decades. He already had adult children, and she wanted to have a baby with him.

She said that several doctors had told her she was anorexic, and she was indeed very, very thin, but I didn't think this diagnosis or label was helpful or true – she was neither interested nor uninterested in food; she simply appeared not to care if she fed herself or not. Sometimes she ate a lot, and other times she went without food for days without noticing. At times she couldn't even remember the last time she had eaten. She also hadn't had a period for years.

This pattern of not knowing what was good for her had been repeated throughout her life. Although she claimed she was happy in her relationship, she didn't convince me. She gave enormously to him and everyone around her but seemed to receive little in return. She'd had an affair with another man earlier and fallen pregnant, but decided against having the baby at a very late stage because she wasn't sure she wanted to be a mother after all. She would regularly visit friends in the country at weekends but almost always describe the experience as a waste of her time as she ended up doing all the cooking and washing-up. She was strangely undemanding of me and of the people around her, and yet from the stories she would tell me it was clear she ultimately felt empty and alone.

At our sessions together, in addition to using needles, I used a very prescriptive form of support by giving her homework, and asking her to eat breakfast every day for three months and keep a diary of this in order to maintain her focus. It felt like teaching a child. As treatment progressed over many months, slowly she opened up and began to talk about her relationship, her friends and her work, and to see what she actually got from these different areas of her life. She started to recognise the people and activities that gave her a feeling of satisfaction and joy and most strikingly began avoiding the people that took her for granted and took advantage of her very sweet and giving nature.

Her periods didn't restart and she didn't gain much weight, but she did conceive again and carried the baby to full term. Her doctor, who had threatened to forcibly send her to a treatment centre for anorexia was amazed at how this stick-thin woman could carry a pregnancy with such ease and grace and produce a healthy well-nourished baby girl. Having the baby seemed to further engage Sarah in the material world. She transformed as she embraced motherhood and developed the art of asking for and receiving help from her friends and properly integrating into the group.

Metal

Metal is the element associated with autumn, the point in the annual cycle where plants are dying and everything is sinking back into the earth. The harvest is stored and anything we don't need should now be swept away. What's left is a very pure, mineral essence, stripped down and compressed much like the gold and diamonds we find buried deep within the earth. When this element is in distress in a person, the colour we see in the face is white, and the timbre of the voice is a weep, like gentle sobbing. The smell is of something rotten, as though the person's pores aren't opening properly and clearing away the waste.

Metal equates to the value of things: our inner and outer riches. The associated organs are the lungs and the colon. The lungs draw in fresh air and represent our ability to take life in, the breath of heaven, keeping us alive and connected. The colon is connected to earth and death and a final rotting-down, and the removal of waste. When metal is in balance we take in freshness and discard the nonsense and extraneous detail of our everyday lives. We know who we are and the value of our unique role in the world, and we also have a natural mechanism to rid ourselves of doubt or derision. Preserving that purity is essential to our well-being, whether it's emptying the rubbish bins or letting go of something hurtful that someone has said to us.

Unsurprisingly, people with a metal imbalance can feel like they live under a dark cloud or are buried in the clutter (often literal) and minutiae of everyday life. They flap around hopelessly, not knowing what they're looking for or how to find it. Physically, they have a tendency towards symptoms related to poor waste removal and can have issues with constipation and diarrhoea. In Chinese medicine the skin is considered to be the third lung which breathes and connects with the outside world, so they may struggle with eczema and psoriasis, have problems breathing fully and deeply, and often suffer from asthma or recurrent bronchial infections.

The primary emotion is grief as though they were living in a void, or caught in a memory of someone or something and unable to move on in the present. The person often looks longingly to another time. A lot of people with a metal imbalance are weighed down with the sense that they are not good enough, and this gets in the way of them completing the task before them. Old baggage and a lack of fresh inspiration drag them down and distract them. They're always looking for something better because they cannot relish the good that's here right now. Nothing ever feels good enough, so they become critical of themselves and others, and this makes them dismissive and cynical. When this element is out of balance in a person who has had problems with fertility, even an embryo can be dismissed on the grounds that it is unlikely to survive.

If you've ever come across that "yeah, life's pointless but let's get on with it anyway" attitude, you may have met someone whose metal is sick.

Metal: a case study

Virginia was at least 20 minutes late for her first appointment, and arrived with a list of excuses. She had chewed nails and laddered tights. As she searched for her medical records in her large handbag, she revealed, among other things, an empty yoghurt carton and a screwdriver.

Even though she wore expensive clothes she looked slightly dishevelled, and the stories that poured out of her mouth were full of gossip, resentment and blame. Everything about her was slightly off-kilter, as if she were completely overwhelmed by her own negativity.

Virginia was 39 and had been with her partner for just over five years. They had never used contraception, had never conceived, and Virginia had given up hope that she would ever get pregnant. She had come for treatment because a friend had insisted that she try. She reluctantly answered my questions and appeared unwilling to entertain any suggestions from me about diet, exercise and so forth. She seemed to have lost faith in everything.

This "experience" of Virginia in the room told me everything I needed to know about how I could help her. No doctor, blood tests or scans, not even Virginia herself could have revealed in words so much to me as she did in this first session. She had been diagnosed by her consultant as having unexplained infertility, but the truth was that she was emotionally and physically a mess.

My job with Virginia was a simple one. I had to help her clean up her act and bring back a sense of hope. Acupuncture treatment is unbelievably effective in a situation like this. There is an acupuncture point on the lung channel called "Meridian Gutter" which, when needled, acts like a broom that brushes through the meridians (the energy pathways), clearing the rubbish from the gutters, the darkened corners, and bringing fresh air and space to every part of the body and mind to reveal the spirit. It sounds bizarre, but with patients like Virginia it can be nothing short of miraculous.

After treatment Virginia was transformed. She arrived on time to her next appointment and said she felt as if an enormous weight had been lifted off her chest and shoulders. She had spent the whole week cleaning her house, without any suggestion from me, her bowels had started to become regular and her joint pain had eased up so much that she didn't need the medication she had been prescribed. She even talked about the possibility of becoming a mother.

After a year she conceived naturally and had a very happy and healthy pregnancy ending with the birth of her daughter, Lily.

Water

Winter is the season of the water element and is the time when everything in nature is still and quiet. Energy and power are hidden and low. Someone with a water imbalance has a blue tinge to their face, and the timbre of their voice is a groan, a weak, strained and monotonous sound, or else it is a relentless deluge. The odour is putrid, like stagnating water which hasn't been moving as it should. Winter was historically a challenging and terrifying time for people as they waited and hoped that their supplies would last until the spring, and the associated emotion is fear.

We all need fear to survive. Fear alerts us to danger and gives us the reflex to stay safe by providing the energy for "fight or flight". Something as simple as crossing the road requires an appropriate amount of fear: healthy caution helps us sum up the risks before we stride out. This automatic reflex that most of us take for granted is often lacking in people with an imbalance in water. These patients sometimes take huge risks, as they can't calculate whether they should be cautious or not. Equally, people with a water imbalance can swing the other way and become abnormally afraid of everyday life. They feel nervous of using new machinery in case something goes wrong, convince themselves that the approaching storm will destroy their home, and even something as simple as coming for an appointment with someone like me can turn into a nail-biting cliff-hanger affair. Many times I have actually jumped myself on approaching a patient for the first time, as they leap to their feet, eyes wide open. They often develop phobias as their underlying fear is projected out on to all kinds of situations.

The bladder and the kidneys are water's associated organs. In Chinese medicine the bladder has a much greater importance than we give it credit for in the West. The bladder doesn't just act as a container for waste water; it also assesses the balance of fluid in the whole body and ensures that the proper reserves are held in the right physical location for the right amount of time. For example, we need fluids in our eyes for lubrication and tears and secretions in our genitals for sexual intercourse. The fluidity and ease of movement throughout the system is dependent on the function of the bladder, while the kidneys control and distribute the fluids and are responsible for the underlying power and energy of the whole body. The kidneys hold our very essence, the core of who we are, and give us our deepest sense of self; our identity in form.

Water, then, is the element that controls the endocrine system, and is instrumental in the regulation of our moods, growth and development, and importantly, sexual function and fertility. People with a causative factor in water often suffer from a low libido and general lethargy, at times even presenting with a history of recurrent miscarriage. Kidney problems affect the distribution of fluids – resulting in symptoms like oedema, swollen ankles or dry eyes. People whose water element and energy have become deficient will experience symptoms of cold and stagnation – feeling inert and clammy to the touch.

Water: a case study

My first consultation with Jen was extraordinary. As she told me about her failure to conceive she became hysterical. I have seen people devastated or depressed about not getting pregnant, but this woman was desperate, crying and wringing her hands.

In the past I used to work more slowly and bear with people's various ways of communicating, but I've become increasingly inclined to cut to the chase when it is obvious that a patient's behaviour is so inappropriate it will slow down the process of working together to get them well, however harsh that sounds. With Jen, I tried to draw her attention to how bizarre this display of emotion was to me and explain that we needed to regroup and try and get some perspective. She fought at first, but in the course of the next hour and a half she calmed down and started talking coherently. This initial display, however, had told me all I needed to know in terms of how to help her.

Jen and her husband already had a child and were trying for a second. He was frequently away on long work trips, and she preferred to stay on her own with her daughter, rarely socialising. She was living a fairly cloistered life in her pretty house with a state-of-the-art security system because she was terrified of the dangers of the world and other people. If her daughter so much as toddled towards the staircase she would pounce, and presumably terrify the child. She existed in a constant state of fear, and had come to think it was perfectly normal. She worried about crime, child abductions, any threat she could dream up. She told me – and herself – that she wasn't a "people person" and that was why she didn't see many people, but all I could see was a personal security system every bit as defensive as the one set up to protect her home. If you had met her in everyday life, you probably wouldn't have noticed this imbalance, because she had structured her life in a manner that allowed her to avoid, for the most part, dealing with the outside world. It was all damage limitation.

Physically, not surprisingly, she was wrung out with adrenaline. She threw herself into the future and imagined her little girl as an only child, alone and in danger without a sibling. It was almost as if this second baby was imagined as a sort of donor child to help the first child live. It had never occurred to Jen that at base she was trying to protect herself from the world of fear she'd created.

The first task I gave her was to get in contact with two old friends she hadn't seen for a long time. She was surprised at first, and then genuinely shocked as she reflected and realised how strangely she'd been behaving. On the back of this awareness she became more and more at peace in herself, and her desperation for a second child transformed into being simply hopeful. She understood that her daughter would be in no greater danger than any other child as a result of being on her own.

All of these case studies demonstrate how one imbalanced element can greatly affect and dominate a person's life and health and cause all kinds of seemingly unrelated problems. The way that we "are" and behave is frequently dismissed or judged as just part of our "personality" rather than seen as useful information about something far more interesting – how we have become unbalanced. We do it to ourselves all the time with language and excuses such as "I can't help it – it's just the way I am", or "I'm just moody, like everyone in my family", or "I'm a very sensitive person". Worse still, we exacerbate the problem by judging others and putting them in a box when we see repetitive behavior or a certain trait, and label them as "touchy", "irritable", "sympathetic", "nervy", or "great fun". Whatever the label, good or bad, it can be unhelpful, fixing a person in a state that he or she has got stuck in. There is no such thing as an "irritable person", an "anxious person", or a "fearful person". We are simply describing someone with certain thoughts, feelings and behaviours that have become so habitual that they have rendered them unable to move appropriately and are unwittingly causing all kinds of knock-on effects, including problems with fertility.

The Five-Element model teaches us to pay close attention to the part of us that is unbalanced and sick, to become aware of the cause, and do all we can to support that weakness, whether through acupuncture, lifestyle changes, breaking old habits or thinking differently, or a combination of all these. By virtue of the interrelationships between all the elements, any kind of change you make for the better will immediately improve your whole system. Successful conception and pregnancy is always a team effort; ask any team coach the secret of success, and he or she will tell you, "Support your weakest player".

Spirit

A few years ago I was treating a woman called Geraldine, who at the age of 39, had decided to have a child on her own. She was having IUI with donor sperm at a clinic in London and had come for a "boost", but it rapidly became clear that she suffered deeply from depression and many small physical complaints. She told me that her younger sister had died when she was four, and her memories of her parents' grief and withdrawal had affected her deeply. She felt they had lost their real connection to her at that time. By her teenage years, she was on course for what she called "dysfunctional relationships" with men who were chaotic and reckless, and she'd started to abuse both alcohol and drugs.

She said that every morning, for as long as she could remember, she'd woken up with a sense of dread so acute that it was like getting a boot in the stomach. By the time she came to see me she had been through

Alcoholics Anonymous and Narcotics Anonymous and was on the straight and narrow, but she was also desperately lonely. She'd lost a lot of friends in giving up alcohol, and was ticking every symptom for clinical depression.

For us humans to function at our optimum and benefit from good overall health, we need the relationship between our body, mind and spirit to be "balanced". Feeling physically unwell, or emotionally flat, depressed, hopeless or stuck, in my experience, is usually the result of an inability to access our "spirit", and thus experience the miracle of being alive.

When I first considered training in Five-Element acupuncture, although fascinated by the theory of the Five Elements per se, I was not completely convinced by the notion or relevance of spirit. It seemed to me at the time a somewhat unnecessary "airy-fairy" adjunct to this system of medicine and its relevance to health and healing as a whole.

In fact, after three long years of study, I fully appreciated the power of spirit as a key to real success only when I started to work with patients and witnessed many surprising outcomes. Although the notion of spirit as an active ingredient in helping you conceive may seem fanciful and mystical, once properly understood, it will start to feel surpri-singly familiar and logical, and most importantly, transformational. Professor JR Worsley helps demystify the idea of spirit in this extract from his book *Is Acupuncture for You?*

A lot of people feel uncomfortable when you mention the word "spirit". They think you are talking about some mystical entity, or are about to embark on some form of religious crusade. Personally, I feel that one of the great tragedies of the modern Western world is that we have forgotten or we ignore the real meaning and importance of the spirit. We claim to be at the peak of a civilisation but we really live in a barbaric age. Surely, if we were just a mind and a body, full stop, we would be nothing more than clever robots. Technology has provided us with machines that are capable of "thinking" and "doing", but what makes a human being a unique and wonderful individual? What gives that essential quality and spark to human life: its experience of ultimate joy, understanding and compassion? The spirit – that is the spirit. But what importance do we attach to it today? I regret to say, hardly any at all.

Ignoring the spirit is the reason for not winning the fight against disease. We are abandoning and neglecting the deepest and most essential part of a person. If the spirit within us is denied, we will not keep in harmony and balance. Thus we will be more susceptible to disease.

The difficulty with defining the spirit, or what is also referred to as the "true self", is that it is beyond thought and words, and so paradoxically the key to understanding it (one of those Chinese contradictions) is accepting that you can't. It's a feeling thing and can only be understood through experience. It's apparent when you feel fully alive – the "goose bumps" moment when the hairs on your neck and arms lift and you feel something way beyond thought. There have been times in my life when nothing has touched me – everything seemed bland and functional – even things that in the past were so exciting. When I am connected with my spirit, living in my "true self", I can feel it. There's an enlivening quality about the spirit: sometimes small and quietly galvanising, other times awesome and overwhelming, but always indescribable in words.

The ancient Chinese had little problem in recognising and feeling the presence of spirit in everyday life. It was essential. This was a culture that knew from bitter experience that to ignore the spirit would be a threat to their own community and its long-term survival. They understood the "oneness" and interconnectedness of all life, and how spirit is the conduit between our inner and outer world: "As within – so without." For example, the warmth and fullness of summer is reflected in the open-hearted fun we enjoy at this time, and nature's activity in spring is mirrored by the hopes and our plans we feel inside. This symbiotic relationship meant communication between the people and their environment was authentic and balanced and facilitated their success as a race. In our relatively safe and modernised world where our survival needs have changed, this natural attribute has been greatly diminished as our minds have taken on the impossible task of providing us with an authentic sense of self and a meaningful direction in life.

The breadth and potential of each human being's life is unfathomable to the human mind. For this reason, sadly, most of us who "think" our way through life access only a fraction of our potential, and for many different reasons limit ourselves to a relatively thin band of experience and suffer as a result. The purpose of acupuncture treatment is to balance our internal world so that we come from the right place – our authentic self. This enables us to have a harmonious, congruent relationship with the world, and opens the door to the full life potential that nature offers us. In turn, we then contribute to the bigger picture of life in our own unique way. It's a beautiful relationship.

During acupuncture treatment this "tuning" is achieved by selecting specific acupuncture points that address the needs of each person, and it is through this provision that balance is attained. The spirit of all the acupuncture points combined tells the story and holds the mystery of life, and reflects the riches of nature and the world we see around us; the potential and capacity of each human experience is no less majestic than the whole of nature itself.

"Spirit Burial Ground", an acupuncture point located on the chest, serves to resurrect the spirit from under the weight of negative thoughts and experiences. On Geraldine it was electric. She woke up feeling hopeful and even happy for the first few days after her treatment, and we focused on keeping her attention on the part of her that was healthy and well, lifting the old sense of dread for longer and longer periods. She realised for the first time that the love she had been looking for all her life was already present inside her. What we tried to do was maintain that profound connection with her true self, her spirit, which had been neglected for so long.

At the Harley Street clinic she was attending she did IUI, and after her third attempt she fell pregnant. She was at peace with the idea of being a single mum and I could see that it was right for her to do this on her own at that time. Just a year after her baby was born, she met a fellow single parent at the park and is now enjoying a warm and loving relationship.

I had a patient called Glen who was suffering from depression and had an extremely low sperm count. As we talked, he came back again and again to the idea that everything was pointless. He couldn't see anything succeeding so he didn't want to begin anything new. If he embarked on one course, he'd quickly find an obstacle and be knocked back to where he'd started.

He was unable to make a single decision. It was a longstanding joke among his friends that he would never spontaneously do anything. Even something as simple as the question of whether or not to take a bottle of wine to dinner foxed him. He drank too much and had previously had a heavy marijuana habit, and although he was undoubtedly talented as a choreographer, he didn't have the fight to try to create any new work, and was bumping along in a job he could manage without pushing himself. His girlfriend was despairing but at the same time accepted that this was "just the way he was", and hoped that a child would make a difference.

Treating an acupuncture point located on the back called "Contracted Muscle" mirrors the moment when a taut bowstring is loosened. I used this point with him to help release the pent-up energy, along with a point called "Spiritual Soul Gate" which, as the name suggests, gives the capacity to experience "spirit fly". The other main point I chose many times for him lies on the gall bladder meridian and is called "Great Mound". This provided Glen with the perspective to see beyond the obstacles he had created in his mind.

Before his treatment, I couldn't coax Glen even to begin to imagine what it would be like to be a father. It took some time to see a difference as his reflex to go straight back to that sunken depression was almost overwhelming, but gradually things changed and he became more sociable and even started going to the gym. He didn't come back for further treatment after a doctor told him his sperm count had improved, so I don't know if they were successful in having a child, but things had certainly begun to shift for him.

Five-Element acupuncture is one of many ways to help balance the relationship between the body, mind and spirit, and from my clinical experience it is highly effective, but one of the simplest ways to maintain and strengthen this balance is to spend time in the natural world. Playing with animals and small children, being outside; in fact, anything that promotes a sense of peace will help, but most importantly you must be fully present in each experience in each given moment. Animals and children don't think too much, and if they do it looks quite painful. My dog looks cute when he's trying to understand my words but I can see how much effort it takes. They exist in the moment, responding to life as it happens, in any way that arises naturally in them.

Some of us are so far removed from the natural world and the blissful innocence of childhood that the only way we can reconnect with our spirit is by experiencing such a monumental crisis that our mind and body – no longer able to cope – quit! Numerous accounts of breakdowns leading to a state of peace and contentment demonstrate that the spirit is always there behind the thinking and the chaos. It's more a case of where we put our attention. We focus on our minds and bodies by thinking and doing all the time – even when we go for a walk, we use this time to cogitate rather than just enjoy being outside and walking.

Put simply – we are more than a body and a mind. The qualitative experience of being human comes from our spirit. We can listen to a piece of music with our ears, we can understand how it is composed with our mind, but the enjoyment and qualitative experience come from our spirit. Fake flowers can look impressive and beautiful; we can see them with our eyes and understand that they look real with our mind. Our spirit, however, is not engaged. Body communicates with body, mind with mind, and spirit with spirit.

By focusing your attention on your spirit, allowing your body and mind to rest, you start the process of aligning your body and mind with your spirit.

Optimising Your Fertility

Most guides to conception come with a list of dos and don'ts about what to eat and how to exercise from day 1 to day 28 of the textbook female cycle, and a list of mainly don'ts for the boys: how much protein for breakfast, 30 minutes' walk a day, sex when your partner ovulates, and absolutely no alcohol. For some people creating the right conditions to have a baby can quickly become a full-time job, and certainly take up a huge amount of their waking day. Many people will do anything to have a baby, understandably, and if they read that it helps to stand on their head they'll do it.

Sally's morning begins at 7am with a pint of water, a handful of vitamin pills and a piece of seaweed on wholemeal toast. Then off to a yoga class with just enough time to get to work at 9am. It's day 14 of her cycle and the ovulation test says "yes" so she makes a quick phone call to John to check he will be home by 7pm (she read somewhere this is the best time for sex as her cervical mucous will be copious at this time). She doesn't like her job and hasn't for over five years, but the maternity benefits are great – so she stays. She pulls herself through the day snacking on nuts that stick in her teeth and annoy her, but she has heard that a regular supply of protein is good for the blood.

Her partner, John, looks at his watch, puts away his phone and lights a cigarette. It's only one a day now but the guilt goes deep. He goes back to his desk and hears his colleagues laughing as they recount the adventures of the stag night he missed the previous Friday night. His new life of abstinence, enforced relaxation and timed sex is taking its toll and he doesn't feel good.

And so it goes on, for many people, for months and even years. This daily regimen is stressful and soul-destroying, changing as each new tip of the week supersedes the last, rewriting the ever-changing formula for how to get pregnant. This process wears people down not only physically and emotionally, but more importantly, spiritually. As faith and hope are slowly undermined by each failed attempt to get pregnant, they dig themselves into a desperate state. People forget who they are, and what they really like. Their relationships suffer dreadfully.

Very often the task in hand also causes people to overlook their real underlying problems: that Sally hates her job – which she spends hours on every day – and John is consumed with guilt and he misses the old, fun life he had before he began trying to be a dad. And all the time, they're trying to fit themselves into a rigid way of life that has nothing to do with them personally, and was dreamt up as a "one size fits all" cure for infertility.

Sometimes when I am treating people, I ask them to do something specific like eat a decent breakfast or get a certain amount of exercise, but it's by no means a militant approach. The most interesting thing for me as a practitioner is to encourage people to get a real sense of who they are and what works for them. Maybe they'd rather parasail once a week than go to the gym every day, or eat oysters simply because they enjoy them and they make them happier than a zinc supplement. If you feel better for a night out, you feel better full stop. Guilt will hardly improve the situation or your health.

This isn't to say that a life of unthinking self-indulgence is the key. The Five-Element approach requires you to step back from everything that is going on in your life and look again through the soft-focus lens of your instinctive self. Without realising it, people in the modern world have slowly slid into a way of living and a mode of thinking that seem normal to them but aren't remotely natural or good for them, and which could be impacting negatively on their fertility.

If someone is living completely out of whack, I recommend that they "reset" their system for three months using an approximation of what's called the

Law of Midday-Midnight, or the Chinese Clock, which I will explain in more detail later. They may not carry every part of it on into their future lives, but some good habits will have been formed in that time, and most importantly, they will have understood when and how they violate what Chinese medicine calls "the natural laws".

Violating Natural Laws

All of us violate natural laws every day of our lives. We ignore hunger when our stomach rumbles, eat when we are thirsty, take a painkiller for a headache when we know we should stop and rest, avoid confrontation when actually that might be a way of moving on in our lives, and deny or delay an instinctive drive to start a family.

Some people are born with incredible innate resources that mean they can get away with pushing against the natural laws and their health. Others might live just as long but have a weak constitution or live in difficult circumstances, and constantly have to bring themselves back to that centre of premium function – bolstering their systems with extra sleep, better food choices, healthy relationships and being more careful with their energy. You need to have a sense of your own limitations as an individual and not expect yourself to be able to cope with the same level of activity as others around you. You may be able to get by with less sleep than them, or you may need more. When you are in touch with your body and needs, you will be better able to judge this.

As we get older we often accept low-grade health as a norm. We feel "tired all the time" but don't connect it with not eating properly or exercising enough, or taking enough breaks from staring at a screen. We get used to being stressed and anxious as the little vices accumulate. We're like the frog in the pot of water, who does not realise that the heat is on underneath, and the temperature is gradually rising.

You wake up tired, so you kick-start yourself with caffeine before heading to a stressful work environment that causes your cortisol levels to soar. You shovel down a sandwich at your desk and barely taste it. More coffee or tea to stave off that dip in the afternoon, and then by the time work is over you're cross-eyed and frayed, so you have a drink to take the edge off. Too many drinks and you sleep badly, wake up tired and begin the cycle all over again. And of course, it's all just "normal".

It's not that we're incapable of feeling as energised and relaxed in our late thirties and early forties as we were in our twenties, it's just that we lose our ability to judge that we are moving further and further out of balance.

Our body has been designed with a perfect clock, so

these good habits are latent in us, so to speak. The trouble is, our heads usually overrule this inner clock, and our lifestyles demand that we stretch it to the utmost. We think we can stay up all night and keep up our usual routine for the following week without any difficulty, and get surprised when we can't. The principle of homeostasis or a natural inclination to swing back into balance applies here too. You stay up till 4am one night, and a couple of days later you will pass out on the sofa at 8pm. Unless we try to override nature with coffee or caffeine drinks, nature will override us.

As much as nature wants us to procreate, its primary aim is for us to simply survive, so it won't put us at risk with reproduction in a stressful environment. Instead it husbands resources and short-changes our reproductive capacity so that the rest of the body can cope with the harsh environment. Many men who present at the clinic with low sperm counts are in high-stress jobs, and are so set in their ways that quitting or coming off that adrenaline is unthinkable to them. Not surprisingly, their bodies are channelling resources away from their reproductive systems. Equally, it is not uncommon for a woman's menstrual cycle to stop completely when the pressure of life gets too much.

The idea that stress affects fertility has now begun to be considered by Western medics too. In May 2011, the scientific journal *Fertility and Sterility* published the results of an experiment by Dr Alice D Domar, a doctor who specialises in helping patients to deal with the trauma of infertility. She studied 100 women who were taking a course of IVF treatment, 50 of whom were also following a "stress management" programme which included cognitive behavioural therapy, learning relaxation techniques and participation in support groups. After the second cycle of IVF, 52 per cent of the women who were being helped and supported conceived, compared to 20 per cent of those who had had no stress-management sessions.

Many major US fertility clinics now offer similar support schemes. Dr Domar told the *New York Times*, "It's not that it's all in your mind. If you're really stressed out the body seems to sense that it's not a good time to get pregnant." This is exactly what I would tell my own patients, although it can be hard to get them to realise that they are seriously stressed. Quite often, when I ask people about their day-to-day lives, they don't spot the contradictions till they are forced to go through each part bit by bit – and discover a chain of cause and effect quite different from what drove them in the first place.

There is a point where nature will not allow us to continue pushing ourselves in this way, the problem manifesting itself usually in the form of physical or emotional symptoms or even a spiritual crisis that tells us we have to stop and look at what is going on in our life and with our health. We need to understand that this symptom offers us the chance to step back and change something, whether it's diet, exercise or a preparedness to be more honest with ourselves.

One woman I treated was head of a major multinational in the UK. She'd conceived three years before, at a time when she was travelling back and forth between London and New York on a regular basis for frequent business meetings. She got off a plane one day and miscarried. She conceived again, and the same thing happened. Shortly after that she split with her partner but in relatively little time found herself in a very happy new relationship. They were both keen to start having children quickly as she was nearing forty, and worried that they wouldn't have much time.

They also bought a new house in the countryside, which, although pleasant and peaceful, was hours outside London. She started getting up early in the morning and kicking off work at 6am with her Blackberry and laptop on the train, which she thought was an efficient way of doing things. She then worked a full day in London and left the office at 7 or 8pm at night. On top of this, she still did transatlantic flights on a frequent basis and shuttled back and forth to Frankfurt, where the company was setting up a new office. She already had a huge amount on her plate when she came for her first appointment.

She wasn't an overtly aggressive person, but there was something jarring to me about the considerable energy that she gave off in the treatment room, as though she was frustrated and wanted me to get on with things. She enjoyed her job and thrived on what she called the stress of it, and in many ways she had the reserves to deal with it, but perhaps not to carry a pregnancy at the same time. It was as if her body had not even acknowledged her pregnancies when they happened – she'd felt no fatigue or morning sickness, but simply ploughed on.

The initial consultation and treatment had an instant effect. I asked her to try to leave work at 5.30pm every day, and to take an hour out of the office every day to do something purely for herself; she chose a Pilates session at a local gym. I never suggested she should change jobs, but a few weeks later she jumped ship after ten years at the multinational and walked straight into a high-powered job with a competitor. She and her partner had given up on conceiving naturally and were looking into travelling abroad to find an egg donor, and she was excited at the thought. She had a three-month fallow period to make the transition between the old job and the new, and it was during this time that to her surprise, she fell pregnant naturally. This time round she experienced the full quota of pregnancy symptoms; she was tired and sick and hungry and needed to give herself time off to relax. It was as though she surrendered to the physical changes for once, instead of letting her head overrule her body.

She could easily have gone on with her busy lifestyle

but in her case, something had to give. There are always going to be people who are physically hardy enough to conceive on such a regimen and thrive on it, even if they're not in their twenties any more. But if you are trying to conceive, and run into problems, particularly those "unexplained" ones, a change of environment for that pregnancy might yield faster results than you'd imagine.

Almost any of us are capable of returning to full health given the right treatment and support. My experience with my patients reinforces my belief and optimism that almost anything is possible when nature is given the chance to do what it is designed to do and we surrender ourselves to its plan.

The Law of Midday-Midnight

Nature has a plan for you! The Owner's Manual was conveniently installed inside you when you were born and provides all the information you need to survive in your given environment and live a healthy, productive life. This is great news for you – providing you remember to refer to it. Sadly most of us do not – not because of apathy or an impatience to get on with life, but largely because we're not aware it actually exists, and even if we are, we prefer to fumble through without it. I, like many people, used to hate instructions, so buying a new electrical appliance or anything that required direction was going to have a successful outcome only if pressing the "START" button was enough.

We typically take the healthy functioning of our bodies and minds for granted until something goes wrong. When we discover we're unable to make a baby it feels as if our body has betrayed us, and yet many of us have been putting our bodies and minds under huge strain for years. Even the people who have technically been looking after themselves more often than not have been abusing their systems without realising it.

I recently visited a friend who was complaining about a plant he had bought from a local shop. "What a rip off. Fifty pounds for a brown stick!" he moaned, and pointed to the skeletal remains of a Ficus tree sitting in his window. I could see the small white plastic label that came with the plant poking out between the brown, crinkly leaves. "It says you shouldn't place it in direct sunlight," I commented helpfully.

Nature has designed us in such a way that every part of us will function at its best when we are in sync with our environment, which is location- and time-sensitive. Our environment is always in a state of change and responds to the rhythms of day and night. The Law of Midday-Midnight is a body, mind and spirit "clock", that runs for a 24-hour cycle, broken down into twelve two-hour periods.

In each of these two-hour periods, one of your ten

organs and two functions that relate to one of the Five Elements benefits from an increased supply of energy – the peak flow. This two-hour period becomes their high point and a window of opportunity for them to function at their optimum. Conversely, the organs or functions at the opposite side of the clock have less energy, they operate less efficiently and experience their low point, a time to rest.

I explained in an earlier chapter how imbalances in the Five Elements are frequently dismissed as personality traits; so too can disturbances in the Chinese Clock give rise to problematic symptoms and behaviour. For example, many people say that they are not "morning people" and accept that half of the working day is written off. Others slump mid-afternoon calling it a "carb crash" and collapse at their desk, and some who are stuck to the sofa at 7pm believe that an evening in front of the TV is all they can manage. Who relishes waking as bright as a button at 3am knowing there's a full day of work ahead? All these symptoms tell us our clock is running out of sync.

The Law of Midday-Midnight teaches us the importance of "rest and play" and to respect the enormous and complex tasks that the organs and functions do for us daily to ensure our general well-being, our reproductive health, and our survival. By ignoring this law we put extra pressure on these "Officials" and our system as a whole. The importance of the "team effort" is again emphasised here as any disturbance at any one period of the clock will immediately have a knock-on effect through the rest of the 24-hour cycle. When you work with nature's time schedule all areas of your health, including your fertility, are greatly improved and your whole system runs in one rhythm like a well-oiled machine. The following description of the Chinese Clock provides an understanding of how our organs and functions work and rest internally, and tells us how, ideally, we should live our lives externally.

The clock is a cycle and so we could start our journey at any point, but the early stirrings of a new day is a good place to begin. Between 3am and 7am, the metal element predominates and the lungs and colon are prioritised. For the first two hours your lungs benefit from the cycle's surge of increased energy, enlarging their capacity, awakening and oxygenating every cell in your body and every corner of your mind. From 5am to 7am the peak flow shifts to the colon, which now has its best function – this is the optimal time to rise, have a bowel movement and release the physical and mental waste of the previous day. You'll remember the metal element is responsible for maintaining the "quality" of your health, and is achieved by the taking-in of fresh air and the release of all waste.

Mavis came to me almost 20 years ago, and at that time was in her mid-forties. Her main complaint was long-term infertility and chronic arthritis in all her major joints. I treated her at the first session and asked her to drink two pints of water every day. She was resistant to the suggestion, claiming that throughout her life she had never drunk water as she had grown up in a remote part of India where they only drank tea and gin! She left, however, saying that she would comply with my request. Two weeks later she arrived at my treatment room looking radiant but concerned. "What have you done to me?" she asked. Reluctantly, she started to describe the events of the previous ten days; how three days after drinking the allotted water she woke at dawn, which was unusual for her, and was compelled to get up, put on her dressing gown and slippers and walk into her garden to sniff the air. This early-morning constitutional in its turn induced severe cramping in her lower abdomen and she'd find she'd then be forced to sit on the toilet where "all this disgusting stuff" would come out of her. On further questioning it became apparent that it had been normal for her to have a bowel movement only every ten days and so this daily excretion was new and quite shocking. Within a month her arthritis had completely gone away and she had her first menstrual bleed in five years.

Nature always gives before it takes. When a child clings to something it should not have, trying to take it away with force creates resistance. Distract the child with the offer of something new and the little treasure will hand over the object with ease. We can see this in the case of metal and all the other elements. When the lungs open and expand to receive the fresh morning air, this relative excess to the colon provides the release to let go. Nature ordains that all waste be removed at this time, and so in good health we empty our bowels, and shower away the waste from our outer lung – our skin.

Not surprisingly, the stomach is king over the next two hours, as the energy moves out of the colon and surges into the earth element, stimulating hunger and providing the energy to digest almost anything. The old saying that you should breakfast like a king and dine like a pauper is apposite. It's very basic – "nature abhors a vacuum" – and as you empty the lower part of your digestive system you refill from the top. You need enough fuel for the day. Would you really set off on a long car journey with no fuel in the tank? Fully satiated, the next stage from 9am to 11am is when the spleen is handed the energy baton and swings into action – transforming your intake into something suitable for both physical and mental consumption and transporting it to every part of you to give the resources to move every muscle and get good thinking and working done.

The heart, imbued with its daily energy charge, rules in the middle of the day, from 11am to 1pm when it is good to relax and begin socialising – work meetings, conversation, joining friends for lunch. The small intestine then steps in to filter and organise from 1pm to 3pm, sorting and clearing the day's new information and deciding what to keep and what to throw away in anticipation of a productive afternoon of work.

Water takes centre stage in late afternoon and early evening between 3pm and 7pm. First the bladder stores and reserves what you will need later. In Western medicine it's just a sack for urine, but in the Chinese system it has the task of making sure you have enough energy for every task – a reservoir. It keeps reserves of fluid throughout your body, for your joints, your digestive system, your sexual excretions and tears. Lots of people experience a dip in energy in late afternoon because their reserves are low, but it should, if you are living by the clock and drinking enough water, be a time when you're feeling an abundance of stored-up energy. The kidneys benefit at 5pm, when the body and mind's reserves are consolidated and you have a heightened experience of your own existence, and a profound sense of your "essential self".

At 7pm the fire element receives its second surge of energy as it enters into the two fire functions that occupy the next four hours. It's a time for the circulation-sex function to come to the fore, a time for relaxation, socialising and sex, and being with other people rather than sitting at home alone. Interestingly, this is the stomach's resting period – when it has the least energy available – and yet most of us have our biggest meal of the day at this time. Is it any wonder our sex lives suffer? The second stage is ruled by the "three heater" or the body's heating engineer, which busily travels around every part of our being, adjusting and correcting the physical and emotional temperature. It brings you down from the heat and activity of the day to a cool, resting state, ready for deep restorative sleep.

The hour of sleep before midnight is important to start the natural rhythm of rest. It is said "an hour before midnight is worth two thereafter". Wood covers this hour, as well as the three after midnight, when first the gall bladder redirects the essential inner activity of regeneration, and then from 1am to 3am the liver steps up to store and detoxify the blood. The liver presides over our deepest sleep and the dreams that help our unconscious make good plans for the next day without the interference of everyday life. "Let me sleep on it," we commonly say when needing time to reflect and access the "vision" of wood and the liver.

What I found charming about the Law of Midday-Midnight when I first learnt about it was that it made me feel I didn't have to be completely in charge of everything. It also made me realise that there is an enormous intelligence at play keeping me alive while I am running around living what I call "my life". In the West we're told we have the freedom to work everything out for ourselves, and sometimes that freedom promotes an arrogance that is counterproductive. In the Chinese Clock your body and organs already know how they will best function, and how to give you the full life experience. If we work with them and follow the natural laws, it all falls into place, and it's less of a struggle. Notice that the Chinese Clock has nothing to say about eating salmon or jogging for 30 minutes a day. There's room for flexibility; you just have to acknowledge that by not working with this "law" you're not doing yourself any favours.

Any opportunity like this to find humility and be

grateful for natural laws and our proper place in the world is a step in the right direction when it comes to conception – a simple moment in nature's work. The human mind is a relatively new phenomenon in the history of our universe, which means it is less well equipped to compete with the ancient Law of Midday-Midnight. Obviously, if you consistently violate natural laws without thinking or compensating for that swing out of kilter, then you will find that your body, mind and spirit will adjust. We are hugely resourceful, but any imbalance puts a huge strain on the system and eventually unease manifests itself in griping health problems, tiredness, gloom or unhappiness.

Many of the people who seek help do so saying that they feel well; but they are generally living in a false reality as the time-bomb of ill health has yet to be revealed. Early warning signals are sent well in advance by nature, sometimes as early as ten or fifteen years; these are the niggling symptoms we get used to, a colour in our face we put down to fatigue, a spate of restless nights we blame on noise, unexplained infertility we cannot understand.

Men v Women

The World Health Organisation figures for global fertility are as follows:

– One in six couples are infertile. In 40 per cent of cases the problem lies with the male, in 40 per cent with the female, 10 per cent with both partners and in the remaining 10 per cent of cases the cause is unknown.

– One in 25 males has a low sperm count and one in 35 is sterile.

There are huge variations in these numbers all over the world, but this breakdown still shows that infertility is a shared problem between men and women.

I have tried to include as many examples of men as possible, because as is clear from statistics, infertility can affect men and women equally. If there are fewer stories centring on men in this book, it's not because they play a lesser role, but simply because they are generally more reluctant to seek help and I have worked with fewer men by far.

Twenty-three years ago when I started working as a psychotherapist, my clients were mainly women and gay men. When I qualified as an acupuncturist the same two groups made up the vast majority of my patients. As I began to get a reputation as a fertility specialist, there were even more women in my practice, although in many cases it was the male half of a couple who needed treatment, and not the female.

We live in a culture where for thousands of years

women have been given sole responsibility for conceiving (or not conceiving) babies, and that mindset still dominates. There are far more fertility procedures that deal with women's bodies than those of men, who are often given a clean bill of health after just one decent sperm test. It's women who congregate at web communities to discuss menstrual cycles and diets, commiserating and bonding, not men, whose feelings about their own infertility are often far more private, though still deeply felt.

The majority of women who come to me still turn up on their own, and continue to have treatment solo. It can be difficult to persuade men to involve themselves because they tend to be more cynical about alternative treatments like acupuncture and psychotherapy, and indeed about seeking help in general. They are also sceptical about spending money on supplements when these treatments seem to offer so few results. If the doctor has said there's nothing wrong with their sperm, they don't see why they need to change anything about their lifestyle. I see men taking their responsibilities as fathers seriously the moment their child is born, but it's rare to see a guy who's on a special diet and working out in order to improve the quality of his sperm and his chances of conception. Generally, a man's attitude is that if his female partner wants to pursue an alternative route of help, she should go ahead, but not drag him into what he sees as women's business. When his partner then turns round and says it would be a good idea for them to have some kind of treatment, he will normally resist.

If one half of a couple makes changes to their life – be it through therapy, acupuncture, a change in diet or any form of self-improvement – it's often the case that this active partner will suddenly make a leap forward and become even more separated from their other half, who then seems left behind and stuck in their existing way of living. I try to encourage both men and women to prevent this kind of thing happening – asking for help and making changes isn't just about getting pregnant, but about improving your quality of life. It seems a shame that only one half of the equation should benefit.

Times have begun to change, and I've seen a steady increase in the number of men seeking help for all kinds of problems, not just infertility. Those men who do plunge in, though, often do it out of a sense of duty to their spouses, and they don't seem to have that same desperate drive as women. Sometimes, buried deep down, are very private feelings about the whole process. Men have to contend with a lot of built-in notions of pride and shame: that they're not *real* men if they can't get their woman pregnant. They're supposed to be nonchalant about the process and sometimes are, to the extent that they get left behind and all but left out. Feeling sidelined, it doesn't seem to occur to them to keep themselves in shape in order to maintain the quality of their sperm. Often I'm shocked when a new male client tells me his age – it can be ten years younger than I would have guessed.

What sometimes makes this worse is the fact that women are usually the first ones to seek help from a professional practitioner like me, or their gynaecologist or their fertility guru and they do this by themselves. Because they're talking about their deepest hopes and fears and the most secret physical and sometimes emotional issues, they rationalise this intimacy by forming quite an intense and personal bond so that the problem of conception becomes more of a project between the woman and the professional than between her and her partner.

Suddenly the fertility expert becomes teacher, best friend and magician all rolled into one. The women throw all their hopes into this one individual and his or her team, making them into their new support system, and stop focusing on their partner and the relationship which should be the very core of their desire to have children. The man is expected to play his part by providing sex and sperm, and after that's over the woman reports back on progress to her real buddy in fertility – the practitioner.

A good example of how men can get lost in the system is evidenced in Michael's story. He originally came to me for a chronic toothache that had been going on for years, only clearing up for brief periods when treated with antibiotics. He was in his mid-thirties, worked in television and lived in south London with his girlfriend Janet and her two sausage dogs – Samson and Delilah. During our first meeting he was absolutely tickled that I was asking him about his childhood when all he wanted was localised pain relief for his tooth. When I moved on to do the physical exam and felt his spine and other areas of his body, he burst into hysterical laughter. "This is mental," he spluttered.

People find it very strange that we take so much time to take a full medical and personal history before addressing any symptom. Michael's, however, was a good example of a situation where a long-term chronic condition like toothache can have a much deeper root, often missed in Western medicine, which tends to focus on the single presenting symptom. If the body is not responding to medication there is likely to be some underlying cause that could also be affecting other areas of a person's general health.

Michael casually mentioned that he and Janet had been trying for a baby for over three years. I asked him if they had had any medical tests for fertility and started to explore what was wrong. Seeing my confusion with what he was telling me, he then confessed that although his sperm results were excellent, he had erectile problems, coupled with severe and very painful eczema around his genitals, to the extent that they rarely had sex and were now considering IVF as a way of bypassing these problems. His acceptance of the situation was courageous in some ways but there was also something rather sad in how a serious condition was simply swept under the carpet because of the availability of medical interventions like IVF. What would have happened prior to the advent of IVF? So, poor Michael now has antibiotics for his tooth, IVF for his impotence, steroid creams for his eczema – what next, I wonder?

Balance "With a Twist"

On Tony and Karen's first visit, it felt as if I was having a consultation with one person. Tony talked for Karen, in language that ran the two of them together. He'd say "When we were last pregnant", or enthuse about the textbook menstrual cycle "we" had had that month. They had been hoping for a child for over five years and in that time "they" had had three miscarriages. As we talked, I realised that the pregnancy had become very much Tony's project, almost to the exclusion of Karen, who seemed happy to let Tony take the reins. She was happy with her job, with Tony and her life, and if it turned out that they were unable to have kids, very unusually, I don't think she saw that as a disaster.

Tony was clearly a very sweet loving man, but to my mind excessively involved in everyone else's lives and readily admitted his nickname was "mummy"! He wanted to look after everyone. He didn't really want to talk about what he did at work; he would rather share the ways he'd helped work colleagues and friends who'd come to him with a problem. He also proudly admitted that he wanted to stay at home with the new baby once it was born, rather than go to work.

He was genuinely a very caring man, and there is nothing wrong with the impulse to care for a baby, to look after people and to be a good friend, but with him it had become such an urgent and all-enveloping need that it seemed to dominate all traditionally masculine aspects of his personality. I think, too, that the flip side of that need to help friends was his need to be helped and supported in return, which had become a kind of projected action. More often than not it's the woman who loses enthusiasm about her career when faced with the challenging issues of infertility and relies on her male partner to keep the show on the road while dealing with this problem.

I referred Karen to one of my colleagues and began working with Tony myself. After a few months there were no great eureka moments, but I did witness a gradual change in the man. As he slowly started to recognise his own needs, his focus drew back a little from his friends and domestic life, and I found him taking on new hobbies and contracts at work with attack and enthusiasm. With his new salary he organised and booked a surprise holiday for himself and Karen, which made him immensely proud. Karen was essentially very well and hadn't needed much treatment, and although neither of them had had any diagnosed problems before they sought help, it was only after that shift and a romantic time away in the Maldives that she got pregnant.

I'm not for a minute saying that men don't make great house-husbands, or that they should never be in touch with their more feminine side. Quite the opposite, as in Chinese medicine the correct balance of yin (female) and yang (male) in every person is the foundation of good health, and this book is essentially about balance. Women are predominantly female and men are predominantly male, but everyone is a blend of the two and this paired dynamic is witnessed in all of life. For example, we see it in the seasons, the silent power of winter moving into the rapid growth in spring and peaking with the full blossoming and heat of summer – considered the more dynamic, male side of the year. The more receptive and female side is witnessed in late summer, producing the harvest and drawing everything back down through the autumn to preserve life through the winter.

Through their observations of the natural world, the ancient Chinese paid particular attention to a dynamic that not only maintained their life but also created new life. They called this natural phenomenon the Law of

Husband and Wife. This law states that in nature, and so in every person, immaterial of their sex, the husband side of the energy must slightly dominate the wife side in order to keep the wheel of life moving in a forward and creative motion. The Five Elements follow the order of the seasons, the life force flowing upwards on the husband side and flowing downwards on the wife side. The husband side comprises water that creates the wood, wood that feeds the fire and fire that produces the earth. The wife side sees fire producing the earth, earth creating the metal, and metal giving form to the water. This is the natural order and so this law states that the husband side must always dominate the wife side.

This statement can make heckles rise in a modern context but we have to remember that when the Chinese were developing this system of medicine the primary focus of life was survival and so each person played to their strengths.

Both the active and receptive forces we see in life are powerful in themselves and essential; don't get blinkered by the Western idea that the active role is somehow better than the receptive. There needs to be a qualitatively greater force on our husband side to initiate life, while there needs to be a qualitatively lesser force on our wife side to draw life back down and conserve it. This is something that must exist in each person and will not necessarily be evident in a relationship. Interestingly, we see this in the body – acupuncturists take the pulse of both wrists, and the left, or husband side, should always be qualitatively stronger.

What the Law of Husband and Wife teaches us is that there is a natural balance of opposites in nature and ourselves. We are all unique and some men are more feminine and some women are more masculine – this is normal. However, when there is a disturbance within the relationships of the Five Elements, we often start to see a disruption to the natural balance within that person; inappropriate behaviour and physical pathologies can develop and appear to become part of the person's make-up. This is not to judge or support stereotypes of men and women but simply to recognise and support a part of the cycle when it is in distress.

This is a very sensitive area for discussion, particularly as the roles of men and women have changed dramatically in the West over the past 100 years. It is evident that high-flying businesswomen and stay-at-home dads can conceive as easily as anyone else, providing these roles are authentic and rooted in a path that naturally unfolds for each person. Some patients I have worked with have taken jobs that were ill suited to their nature; they pursue a certain career to satisfy other people's expectations, stereotypical roles, and to prove something to themselves. This choice comes at a cost, as going against our nature will inevitably produce symptoms of some kind to let us know we are taking the wrong path.

Tony did not fundamentally change as a result of treatment – he remained a kind, sweet person, and there was certainly no chance of him turning into a red-blooded alpha stud – why should he? The only change was his care and concern over becoming a father became more appropriate and substantial, and rather than just talk and talk, he started to walk the walk with real integrity and then found success.

Relationships

I am often asked about the importance of "the relationship" when it comes to conception. Is it more likely to happen when we are engaged in a healthy, happy wholesome one, or is it irrelevant? I really don't know. What I have noticed over the years is that happy couples get pregnant, feuding partners get pregnant, single people get pregnant; equally, these same groups don't get pregnant. But I don't think this is an issue that should be ignored.

Relationships are wonderful and inevitable but they can also be messy; in fact, quite ugly at times, and just as the weather will change outside your window, one moment calm, the next moment stormy, so will the dynamic between the people we see inside. It is simply not true that fertility is dependent on a Waltons-esque environment. Babies are conceived in all kinds of relationships – loving and warm, cold and indifferent, bullying and victimising – some even as a result of rape, sadly, so we must observe and accept this fact and look further for truth.

One notable and interesting observation I have made is that the people who have struggled to conceive and have then gone on to be successful seem to be the ones who have significantly improved their relationship with their "self", and their general health – regardless of whether they are coupled up or not. Of course, being in a healthy relationship rather than an unhealthy one is important to our overall well-being, but a relationship itself does not seem to be essential when hoping to conceive. If pushed for an answer, I would say that authenticity is the key. Being in an unsatisfactory relationship is not a problem as long as you admit it to yourself and accept it for what it is. However, deluding yourself that you are living a fairytale romance that doesn't actually deliver may have a negative impact on you and your health and thereby your fertility too.

As fertility increasingly comes under the microscope of Western science, the "department" approach to health and healing tends to dominate in any investigation. Is there a problem with the woman's reproductive organs? Is there a problem with the man's sperm? How are the hormone levels? How are the mechanics of the tubes? This approach to treating fertility is medically brilliant, but it is also segregated and clinical, rather than inclusive. Because of the sheer stress of the process, it can separate the long-suffering couple even more and create or exacerbate problems in the relationship. Along with all the emotional difficulties of trying to make a baby there are also logistical issues that can get in the way which, unless addressed, can waste weeks or even years of valuable time as well as thousands of pounds.

A woman I treated when I first started practising came in for help with unexplained infertility as she was about to get married to her long-term boyfriend and wanted to have a baby as soon as possible. There was clearly an issue in the relationship, and I had only been treating her for three or four sessions when she surprised me by saying that she'd realised that she was on entirely the wrong track in her life. I'd encouraged her to be honest with herself and me about her feelings, and to connect with what really felt right to her, and she had come to realise that not only was she with the wrong man, but the wrong sex altogether. She had always felt drawn to women, but had ignored this instinct because it didn't fit into the pattern of life that was expected of her. She split from her boyfriend soon afterwards and almost immediately plunged into a relationship with a woman, and had a child with donor sperm provided by a close friend. She has been so happy since that she counts her blessings and sends me a Rosh Hashanah card to say thank you every year.

Two other gay women I treat who are using donor sperm have been told by the clinic they are attending that they are not allowed to get pregnant at the same time because they are in a committed relationship. This "now it's your turn" approach has caused all kinds of stress and competitiveness between them, especially as they are both in their early forties and feel under enormous time pressure to have a child.

There are a tremendous variety of people struggling with fertility issues, each with their own characters and individualities and quirks, and I've seen unlikely matches that worked and "ideal" relationships that turned out to be painful and complicated.

Mike and Francesca were the perfect couple. I met them together for the first session, and immediately found them charming and well presented. As we chatted, they took it in turns to lead the conversation. They called each other dear and told they had regular sex. They'd met at exactly the "right" time for their careers and had a lovely house in west London with its own gym, where they worked out side by side every morning before going to their workplaces, where they were each on track for excellent careers in competitive industries. They had one "perfect" child, and wanted to have another, but for three years nothing had happened and, after receiving a clean bill of reproductive health from their doctors they had come to see me. Why weren't they able to conceive again?

If anything disturbed the perfect impression they gave, it was an absence of something at the heart of the relationship. They were just neutral. Not angry, not happy, not sad. Their desire for a second child was the only exceptional thing about their emotions and even then, it was a very tidy sentiment.

When I saw Francesca for a treatment on her own, something else started to emerge. She was very dismissive of everything, worst of all herself. I'd ask her about what she'd done that week and she'd begin, "I read this book the other day..." and then, out of the side of her mouth, add, "Tssch, like I read." This tic carried over into everything. It was as though she had an imaginary friend to whom she was saying what she really thought, and all of it was self-deprecating, and she was oblivious to how strange it was.

For two or three months I didn't feel like I was getting anywhere with her, and then she suddenly let slip that every time she got her period she would feel so wretched that she would almost want to harm herself. This confession turned out to be her big breakthrough.

The first thing that happened was that her previously clockwork menstrual cycle broke down, and suddenly she was having a period after three weeks, or after five weeks, and then three again and then nearly six. She was freaked out by the change, and it seemed to bring a trail of chaos into her and her husband's well-ordered lives.

They started coming to appointments talking about arguments they'd had with each other, with their friends, with their parents, anyone whom they'd confronted over something. When she told me what had happened that week, the stories were about arguments and fallings-out, but they were now animated and full of life, and she had no time to add a self-deprecating aside. She complained about Mike and the way he'd behaved on holiday. She was furious with her father over some dispute about money. Everything the couple had brushed under the carpet before now got an airing as they argued over their most crucial beliefs. Their perfect façade was replaced with something more passionate and vital. The treatment they got at the clinic messed them up thoroughly, but it also brought them to life. That neutral emptiness gave way to all sorts of feelings and in the midst of all the chaos, to everyone's astonishment, Francesca finally conceived.

The pregnancy was difficult. Francesca had terrible morning sickness and needed to take a lot of time off work. At the same time Mike was promoted and moved to a new office with a longer commute from home. He would leave the house at 6am and rarely be home before 9pm. Francesca continued to struggle well into her second trimester, until one morning she received an anonymous phone call from someone telling her that her husband was having an affair. Devastated, she called me for an appointment, arrived at the clinic and completely broke down. Rather than be angry with Mike she expressed complete disgust for herself, to such a point that I really thought she might leave and take her own life. The intensity of her grief was profound and there was nothing I could do other than hold her hand as she descended into a deep pit of self-loathing. And then, suddenly, it was over. She looked up at me through swollen eyes and said she was going to be OK.

Francesca's sickness disappeared soon after that and the rest of her pregnancy was as normal as anyone could expect. Mike apologised for his indiscretion and it seemed that through this enormous shake-up of their perfect life, they found a point of balance, having swung hand in hand from one extreme of the pendulum to the other.

I love a happy ending as much as anyone, but let's not be fooled by the romantic idyll of couples who find all the answers by simply forming a magical union; relationships take work. This story might suggest that by allowing the natural chaos of life to enter their artificially perfect world, a window of opportunity was opened for new life to begin. Maybe – but from my experience it is very important not to get too hung up on the quality of the relationship as an entity in itself, but to look instead at the individuals that make up the couple.

I have come to recognise that the enduring relationships with the real happy endings are the ones where each person takes complete responsibility for themselves, independently of the relationship. Healthy relationships grow when the individuals in them each do whatever it takes to be well, regardless of the outcome. Mike and Francesca had obviously papered over their own personal cracks when they first met and were very pleased with the great joint result, until it fell apart.

Sometimes the social pressure driven by the "biological clock" theory makes people panic into relationships that they know in their hearts aren't right for them. I treated a woman called Molly who had found a nice boyfriend called Declan through internet dating in her late thirties, and after months of dating happily, they decided to get married. They'd both specified in their online ads that they wanted to have children, and so they began trying after the wedding, but there were no results after a year.

When she saw me for the initial consultation she told me that she was depressed because she had been unable to conceive, but when I asked her about Declan, she'd just shrug and say he was fine – all right. They hadn't been together for that long but she didn't sound excited about the man – there was no mention of what he did, what he said, all those things that someone in love will tell you, unselfconsciously, when they're smitten.

Declan had moved into her flat, and after a while the basement flat directly below it came up for sale. She wanted to buy it and knock the two apartments together, but found that instead of reaching for this chance for a family home, Declan had simply given up his job and was quite happy on the sofa being supported by her. Had she become pregnant at this point, who knows what would have happened, but instead she just grew more miserable. I began to push her to see if she really cared so deeply for Declan that she could overcome this, and whether he really was the right person. After a lot of tears, she confessed she had rejected many partners along the way and had been holding out for the love of her life, and now at almost 40 even this one didn't make the grade. She ended the relationship and stopped treatment. I'd sensed before she left that it was deep down a relief for her to escape this sanctioned partnership that she'd tried to make work, but the knowledge that it would take her longer to have a child hurt her more than the loss of Declan.

Ending a relationship when you know time is running out can be one of the most painful experiences of all, and the agony is not only because the chances of becoming a parent have decreased, but also because we insist on believing the cultural myth that someone else is meant to make us happy. In Molly's case the rude awakening was a blessing in disguise as she could easily have become completely comatose and compromised her own values, and the dream almost certainly would have turned into a nightmare. Our culture pumps out constant messages that support this flawed idea that we need a relationship – that special someone who will bring us love. What we fail to recognise is that only we can make ourselves feel truly complete.

One couple I saw had had one child and were trying for a second. The wife made every effort to appear warm and full of life and love, but her husband would sit next to her and contradict and criticise every second thing she said. He was sarcastic and made demeaning jokes which she simply laughed off. The contrast between the two of them was marked. They had been through nine rounds of IVF and technically there was no reason why they should not have another child, but it was difficult to keep their treatment on track. He lost interest in acupuncture after a few sessions and there was little change in her, as she had, I think, chosen to maintain her own fantasy about what she described as a "wonderful" relationship. The dynamic between them was so inert and cold that even though, as I have said, I don't believe you need love to make a baby, I couldn't imagine them being successful again.

Both the members in this particular partnership seemed to have lost touch with their authentic selves. As much as we enjoy believing someone else will bring us love, no one out there is capable of loving you as much as you love your Self, so the starting point for all relationships begins at home with you. You loving yourself really means that the generation of love happens *within* you – it is a self-sustaining dynamic not dependent on anything outside of you. It is also worth remembering the Taoist philosophy that teaches us the law of cause and effect; you are the cause, and your life is the effect. Relationships with other humans are the *effect* of how we feel about ourselves. What we love in other people tells what we would like for ourselves, and what we deplore in others is inevitably something negative lurking in us.

When we are wishing to have children and it doesn't happen, we are driven to do all we can to get the picture right and create the best environment. And yes, a good relationship can be part of that picture; but a relationship with someone else is ultimately incidental. The most potent relationship, when it comes to fertility, is the one that you have with yourself.

Bigger Relationships

Healthy human beings enjoy other human beings. We are sentient, sociable, loving creatures blessed with an enormous emotional capacity to love and to be loved.

The majority of us no longer live in a society where the extended family provides "in-house" security, love and support. Families are often spread over many miles, even continents, and may have little or no contact with each other. In the face of childlessness, a common response is to see it as a secret problem, something to be dealt with alone.

A young couple, Peter and Judy, came to me at the end of their fifth year of trying for a child. They were both very stressed and exhausted, having just completed their seventh round of IVF. Every attempt had failed and they were desperate. The most incredible part of their story was that in the five years of hoping to become parents they had not told anyone else about the gruelling process they were going through. Judy worked as a graphic artist and Peter worked for a television news channel. They were both in their mid-thirties and had regular contact with their families and appeared to have a wide social network.

They seemed perplexed that I was so surprised at their need for privacy. When I asked how it felt to keep such a secret, they became defensive and told me clearly that it was a personal issue and "no one's business!" I was curious and pursued my questioning by asking what they told people who asked them if they planned to have children. Judy's rehearsed response was: "No, we don't like children; we are more interested in our careers."

I felt this shroud of secrecy around the issue was intense, almost shocking and had become habitual. When Judy was undergoing IVF she had to visit the clinic daily for blood tests and would tell her work colleagues she was doing a course to learn a new computer programme. When they were invited to parties where they knew there would be children, including their own nephews and nieces, they would intentionally avoid them in an effort to support the story that they had no interest in becoming parents.

It was painful to hear how thwarted their life had become. On the surface they were two successful people in a loving relationship and had everything they could dream of, but underneath they were broken and desperate, bound by their lies and living in the shadow of their secret.

"I don't want sympathy!" Judy barked at me as I suggested it might be helpful to share with someone. "No one understands. All of my siblings have children. How could they help with our situation?" Judy had all the answers. Unconsciously or even consciously, she was trying to exert control over a situation where she had no control. She apparently knew exactly how her family, friends and work colleagues would react if they knew. "They would be embarrassed and not know what to say, so why bother?"

Their response might have been exactly as Judy anticipated, but what she and Peter seemed not to realise was that in five short years they had moved from an open, honest relationship with the people around them to a closed and dishonest one that was causing a great deal of pain.

When I suggested this could be part of the problem they were, understandably, not convinced. They had heard that acupuncture could help increase fertility, so they wanted needles and results, not whacky suggestions. I treated Judy for almost two months and in that time there were some improvements in her health and general well-being, but there was still something in the way, evident in her constant, underlying anxiety and near pathological fear of family gatherings.

Infertility can be a lonely journey. Often the responses of other people are unsympathetic or tactless. One client who was undergoing IVF for a second child had just had over 20 embryos transferred into her uterus and none of them had implanted. When she was told by a stranger that she was wrong not to have had a second child because "only children are a lot of what's wrong with this world", she looked at her healthy, happy son and wondered what this person could possibly hate about him.

Given these negative responses, it is not surprising that fertility problems are often kept a secret from others; some people carry a deep sense of worthlessness and shame. These responses are usually a result of ignorance as much as insensitivity, which is a symptom of the same problem. The truth is we are here together, trying to get along with each other and share human experience. Our sense of separation from each other is something we choose to believe in. In reality we are totally dependent and interdependent on each other.

Secrets may be hidden because they are of great value and must be preserved, or because they are shameful and painful. For the most part they just need the light of day. "A problem shared is a problem halved", and if we can find the right person to share our secret or problem, the simple relaying of the information can be enough to effect a significant change in us. It didn't help Judy to tell me her "secret". I was a professional person who would support her through this time but it meant nothing to her that I knew what she was going through.

Then, much to my amazement, Judy came to a session one day and told me that she had finally announced to her whole family the truth of their "unexplained infertility". She felt like a different person and her family had turned out to be supportive in a way that she had never imagined possible. When I asked her why she told them she said that she had no choice, she needed their help; the words had just suddenly come out.

Judy and Peter re-engaged with their families and in particular the nephews and nieces in a way that had felt impossible before, and now that the "strategy" was in shreds, found they were free to get on with life and enjoy what was on offer to them. A year or so later, during an extended summer holiday spent with Peter's brother, wife and two young children, Judy conceived naturally and now has two little girls of her own.

Being around people is good for us. Being open and honest about both our failures and our triumphs is healthy and normal and gives us the kind of freedom we witness in nature. There is day and there is night, sometimes things go well and sometimes not so well. This is the normal healthy balance that nature teaches us. We can also learn a lot from the experiences of others. One patient, Polly, spoke of her relief when she found another mum at the playgroup who had had difficulty conceiving a second child. Another, Martin, said it was great to talk to friends who had adopted children when he and his wife were considering what to do next.

Asking for help takes humility and courage, but the very act of asking has the power to change a stifled and stuck situation. Sometimes we actually forget to ask; we make the decision that we want something and we employ our will and set about getting it. However, the simple act of asking with all your heart for something that matters to you is enough, the right course of action will follow. It is gentle and easy and usually works. Some call it prayer. Whatever name you wish to give it, just don't forget to ask.

Sometimes being open isn't so much about revealing your true feelings to others, but rather about revealing underlying tension. I met a young woman who was fairly newly married and had been trying to get pregnant for eighteen months. Yet again, she was a case of "unexplained infertility". Neither she nor her husband had any health problems and they were still in their twenties. I asked her why she thought she couldn't conceive and she said she had no idea.

I began to treat her and we chatted during the consultation about her life and how she felt. She mentioned that she had problems with her in-laws, which her husband wasn't sympathetic to. This seemed like a common enough problem, but when I found out a little more I understood why it was disturbing her so much.

She was white and her husband was black, and although his family had been sweet to her, she was struck by a sense of hostility emanating from them. She tried to talk to her husband about it, but he said she was just being paranoid. The in-laws were very polite and said that the couple were welcome to stay at their home, but she couldn't face it. "There was something about the way the wedding was organised," she told me, "as though they were trying to keep people separate."

When her mother-in-law phoned and talked to her husband, he would barely be off the phone before she would ask him if his mother had asked about her, and they rowed frequently about it. He felt that she was rejecting his family for no reason, and she was haunted by the idea that not only did her in-laws secretly resent her, but her husband didn't really love her either. She wanted to be with him, but her instincts were telling her that she wasn't welcome within his family and that she was pushing him away by her lack of trust.

I found her so wrought up that I suggested one day that she openly ask her in-laws if they had a problem with her. The next time I saw her, she told me she'd gritted her teeth and gone to his parents, proud black British people, and they'd assured her that no, they had no problem with her at all.

Now the tension really began to build up. Her husband was angry that she'd effectively accused his parents of racism; his family were rattled by her claim. In the end it all came to a head when she was talking with her sister-in-law, who broke the family silence and admitted that yes, it was true, the family had been uncomfortable with having a white daughter-in-law.

For a while the air was thick with accusations and hurt feelings as everyone finally came clean. Her husband was nonplussed. Her in-laws were embarrassed now that their true feelings had been revealed. Then, suddenly, the storm cleared and everyone was strangely relieved that the big secret was out in the open. Instead of the family splitting at the seams and estranging the young couple, or their relationship collapsing under the strain, the whole lot of them set out into a new future as a family. There were a few wobbles, but two months on, she conceived her first child.

We like to believe that we know what is going on around us. We think that people only know what we choose to tell them and we limit our understanding of others to what they have chosen to tell us. It keeps life simple and safe. And on the odd occasion when people are brave enough to challenge us on what they see as our insensitivity to them, we defensively shoot back, "But you should have told me". The truth is that we are communicating on many conscious and unconscious levels and collecting enormous amounts of verbal and non-verbal information all the time. In fact, the majority of the information that comes out of our mouths is so flawed and inconsistent that we would be better to shut up completely if we really wanted to be understood.

These two stories of how honest, open, loving communication transformed lurking tension and menace and possibly opened the path to conception, remind us of the intelligence of the natural world. New life is born out of appropriate conditions dictated by natural laws. A code of deceit and manipulation and the stress that that combination produces in the body is no different from soil that has been polluted by toxic chemicals – highly unlikely to foster the germination of a seed.

Love

Love is a frequency. We are just like a radio receiver that can receive energy and turn it into sound, and a transmitter that can produce sound and send it out as energy. Love has its own vibration and is rooted in what

I have been describing as spirit. We cannot experience love in our heads, and as brilliant as the human mind is, it is just not designed to tune in. The mind works at the level of thought rooted in the physical, and is there to interpret our experience but it is not the experience itself. It is really important to understand this and to recognise the difference; otherwise we get ourselves into all kinds of confusion.

For the ancient Chinese, it was simple: "love" was life itself. The gift of this planet, the rising of the sun, the changing seasons, even one's own existence: everything natural was a state of love. Love was seen as the active part of life that powered evolution and was benevolent in every way. The creation in spring and the destruction in autumn – the essential balance of these two seasons that turned each year and maintained life – was seen as loving. When we observe nature, we see the creative cycle of the elements and how each element is created from the unconditional love-thrust of the previous element, the original mother/child relationship. By observing how nature creates a cycle that is so absolutely loving, giving and effortlessly flowing, we understand what occurs within us – not because of us, but despite us.

Love is about acceptance and humility. The acceptance of ourselves, of the laws of nature, of the situation we find ourselves in, our friends, our lovers or partners and children. If we accept others as they are and take full responsibility for how we feel about them, regardless of what they do, say or believe, we enter into a loving state – something which takes maturity and is healing and life-enhancing.

On the other hand, the comparatively unseasoned states of "falling in love" and "falling pregnant" are involuntary acts that can catch us off guard at any time. As I have said, I don't think love is a prerequisite for making babies. Certainly, within our current medical approach to fertility, love does not figure at all. Conception is largely seen as a biological phenomenon that sits apart from any emotional influence. Never the less, love clearly has a role to play. Are we more fertile, for instance, when we are in love? Are we potentially disadvantaged if we are trying to conceive and love is not in the picture?

Why do we fall in love and, having "fallen", why is it that we resurface as the honeymoon phase comes to an end? The generally accepted explanation of what happens when we fall in love is that we return to a very innocent and natural state. The state we were in around the time that we were born and shortly after, when we were almost pure consciousness. With our sense organs only just beginning to develop, our only real experience was of being "at one" with everything. We merged into everything around us – we had no boundaries. We couldn't differentiate ourselves from our cot, our mother's arms, our location; we were simply an ecstatic bundle of energy and form. In this precognitive state, providing we were given what we needed, our response to the world was spontaneous and completely unselfconscious.

As we developed we became aware that everything and everyone was separate in the world of form. This included our new-found thoughts and labels that named our separation. We realised that everything has a name – we have a name; that we have two arms and a head and that our parents are separate entities from us. What came with this discovery was the loss of that original experience of being fully integrated with everything, that sense of oneness. Our love of babies and the reason that humans enjoy being with them is that their innocence, their newness and fragile state, taps into something we love and remember, our non-material self; our spirit. When we fall in love the self-created ego cracks, our boundaries are loosed and we experience a return to pure being – no judgments, no preferences – and our existence is eternal and blissful.

When we are in this trance-like state, every part of us functions at its optimum, including our fertility. Falling in love fast-tracks you to a place where everything seems possible and is the perfect state for self-abandonment and conception – it also brings the bonus of a greater frequency of sexual activity.

If you are no longer "in love", be assured that this fall from grace is completely normal as the honeymoon period wanes. The relatively brief window of experiencing the blissful oneness of life feels like an invitation by nature for us to blend and merge. Being in love is a relatively artificial and temporary state that changes our perceptions, and can feel like the experience of taking drugs that raise you up and bring you down. How many of us didn't notice our lover's annoying habits when floating on cloud nine; how he slightly hunches when he walks and she doesn't shave her legs? As the ego boundaries click back into place, so come the judgments, along with the critical mind to re-establish separation, and the inevitable question – where did my soulmate go? At this point, hopefully, the "mature" adult steps in, whose heart and mind find compromise, and accepts the other person for who they are, and embraces every part of them with an appropriate and sustainable love.

My patient Anna was a great teacher for me. At our first meeting her physical beauty and her strong presence immediately filled the treatment room and for a few moments I was completely thrown. When she spoke she locked eyes with me and lacked any self-consciousness as she told me she wanted to have a baby but needed to find a partner first. In the next breath she asked me if I was married. I smiled nervously and chose to change the subject by asking another question; she looked at me suspiciously and folded her arms. Her bold and intimidating style was seductive but it also felt aggressive to me and made me cautious.

The nature of the rapport between the practitioner and the patient is crucial to success in diagnosis and treatment. The relationship is professional but is also dependent on a certain openness and transparency which must be managed by the practitioner. This fine balance can be hard to achieve, particularly when the patient has the skills to cut through the professional veneer. Anna was a master and the first patient to really wobble me. I already felt on the back foot and I could feel myself scrabbling to find my ground. "Why won't you tell me if you are married?" she asked. "It's a simple question." I finally gave in and confessed that I was single, but that wasn't enough. "Why?" she asked defiantly. I managed to find my way back to centre and conduct the rest of the consultation, but she was out to test me, and she was good.

Anna told me she was depressed. She was 36, had a very successful career in public relations and was adored by a string of men who would do anything for her but she said she hadn't found "the one". When she described these platonic relationships, she was effusive and generous in her praise of these men and reeled off the holidays and gifts they had bought for her, but it seemed strange to me that none of these "wonderful" men had made the grade, and that they persisted, surely knowing that they were never going to get what they wanted. Two of them had been "courting" her for over ten years. There was something that Anna was doing that kept them all dangling.

As our sessions together continued I started to feel a disconcerting push/pull dynamic between us, and needed to remind myself that I did not have to feel responsible for her happiness – but I did. This was troubling for me but also a very interesting challenge as I had to presume that whatever she was managing to induce in me was the same as for all the other men in her life. I never knew how she would be with me; sometimes sweet and affectionate and at other times cold and shrill, making completely unreasonable demands. She tested every boundary I created, pushing me and seeing if she could cross it; she knew my weak spot and would go for it like a shark to blood.

After she left I couldn't help wondering if she had found the perfect challenge in me – unavailable as a partner, unavailable as a lover. Anna wasn't just having trouble with self-love and finding a partner; she now wanted a partner that wasn't allowed. It's possible that inappropriately going after what she couldn't have was a way of denying herself the chance of having a child, saving herself from having to enter into any emotional intimacy with anyone at all.

She said she felt "unloved" and alone and yet it sounded as if she knew half of London and had possibly the most feverish social life that any one person could handle. She was unable to benefit from all the love around her and she was so distrustful of her relationships that she was caught in a love/hate dynamic with everyone. Just when I thought I had totally upset her and would never see her again, she would return with flowers and a card. It was painful to see how she struggled, how hard she worked to manage these countless relationships with people and ultimately, how none of them gave her what she needed.

Anna is a great example of someone who possibly either didn't get the love she needed as a child or was given no boundaries. But more importantly, she didn't know how to generate love for herself. She just couldn't be alone. She was always on the phone, always planning the next visit to someone, somewhere. She also believed that once she found the right man and had children of her own she would feel complete. This is part of that Western myth that deludes so many of us. As I said before, there is no guarantee that anything out there will ever truly bring you love and peace.

Anna stopped having treatment when I confessed, after many months without much progress, and with great relief, that I wasn't sure how I could help her. Working with her had brought up many issues for me as a practitioner. She came to me to find a partner and get pregnant, and even though I try my best not to collude with patients' desires, I found it very hard to keep the focus on where I felt Anna was really struggling.

She was a kind, loving and generous person whose spirit shone so brightly you couldn't help but be rather mesmerised by her, but she had to find a way to be self-sustaining and generate love for *herself*.

Love is the universal mix, the great creator and binder of all life, and is present and available to us at all times. If we are unloving, or feel unloved, then either we have lost our connection with the source, or we have taken the misguided step of thinking we could do it alone. The ancient Chinese had a sophisticated and allegorical understanding of how love manifests in humans. The "Utmost Source" – an acupuncture point on the heart meridian – receives the source of love, the "mandate of heaven". This raw essence of heavenly lore is then transformed by our own little love factory, the circulation-sex function, to generate unconditional love for ourself and others.

What this ancient wisdom teaches us is that we as individuals are the creators of love in our life; we are love. Just as our Western culture has spun us the myth about relationships, so too it tells us that love and happiness are to be found outside of ourselves. We are led to believe that we are damaged if we were unloved by our parents, tragic and pitied if we never find a loving mate, and useless and lonely if we fail to have kids. The stakes are high when we buy into this myth, which produces all kinds of neurotic behaviour that can only be described as madness when we look at the lengths to which we will go to chase this elusive love and joy. Those of us who have had enough reluctantly turn our backs on love and call it a day.

Despite all of Anna's difficulties and internal conflicts, two years after we abandoned working together she returned to me with an acute case of morning sickness. She had accepted a marriage proposal from one of her more ardent suitors the previous year and was now four months pregnant.

Do I believe that love will help facilitate conception? Yes, absolutely, but it is not necessarily the romantic love you might have been expecting.

Sex

When talking about love and relationships, it's impossible not to bring up the question of physical passion. When people start out in relationships they have sex in what you might call a normal fashion – in other words, when they feel like it. They want one another, they want to see the physical response of the partnership they're building, and they generate a huge amount of passion.

Lots of couples now leave years between meeting and settling down and finally having babies. When they have difficulty conceiving, it's often the (unspoken) case that their sex life has settled into something comfortable and comforting and a little routine, or worse, it is practically non-existent. Often when couples set up their campaign for conception they mark out a timetable for sex in this or that margin around this or that fertile period. Later along the fertility conveyor belt, they start scheduling sex for strict periods of time around the woman's ovulation, using graph paper and thermometers to stimulate it rather than, say, a sudden, sexy inspiration. It strips all that primitive energy from straightforwardly fancying someone and doing something about it on the spot.

You don't just lose lust and pleasure with scheduled sex, but also intimacy. Little by little the whole process is dehumanised, and the relationship is undermined. I often first see people when they've been on one of these regimens for two or three years, and they're so focused on having a baby that they haven't even noticed what's happened; they assume that as soon as the woman conceives their old love life will just slip back into place without a hitch.

It's easy for all of us to forget the mysterious and exciting time of our pubescent sexual awakening, the innocence of child's play eclipsed by the rising serpent within, transforming us and our playmates into sexual beings and objects of desire. The vital potency of this time is hard to maintain beyond our teenage years and early twenties, particularly if our sexual activity is focused around one partner. But there is no doubt that the dynamism of this early sexual arousal carries the energetic charge designed by nature to ensure the survival of our species – desire more often than not overwhelming rational thought.

In modern society, of course, the excitement of our sexual awakening is overshadowed and blighted for many by the ever-present "fear" of getting pregnant. As Anita explains:

I don't think I'm alone in having had a complete fear and horror of getting pregnant drummed into me throughout my teenage years. A pregnancy would ruin my entire existence, stop me from completing my education, ruin my parents' reputation, drive me to a backstreet abortionist and possible death – it really was the worst thing that could happen. Consequently, many of my generation thought that rabid sperm lurked everywhere, just waiting to catch us unawares and get us pregnant – we all knew that it only took one!

So I went on the pill, used Dutch caps, condoms and coils, determined not to be part of the tragic teenage mum statistic, and tried to dissociate sex from procreation. I always thought that without these magical safeguards I would be pregnant in minutes.

Years passed and I found myself at thirty wanting a baby. I had gathered the husband, the house and all the trappings that were required to provide for the anticipated bundle of joy, and thought that all I needed to do was stop taking the pill and bingo! That's not exactly the way it played out. My four years of unexplained infertility left me feeling a complete and utter failure, at times suicidal, worthless, bitter, twisted and angry with the world. I couldn't understand why something I had tried so hard to avoid (like a disease) was now eluding me, and why everyone else – and people without my advantages – could apparently do it easily.

The self-loathing I was filled with every time my period started was horrible and must have been equally miserable for my husband. I lost all interest in sex unless it was the right time of the month while feeling the whole time that my husband should leave me and find a "proper" woman and that all my other achievements counted for nothing. I was incapable of seeing any joy in my life that wasn't associated with getting pregnant.

When you have had this kind of experience it is hard to find spontaneous desire and passion – your mind has already been primed to harbour negative messages around sex. Every experience we have in life is recorded by the mind and immediately turned into memory. Memory, much like old photos that remind us of something in the past, cannot hold the spirit and freshness of the present moment. So when we engage in sexual activity, only because it is the right time of the month, and with the same person in the same bed in the same way, even though the event is fresh and new, our mind can trump the experience by playing out a memory, dull and void of life. The mind is so powerful that our partner could transform completely before our eyes and we would barely notice the change as the old tape keeps playing in our mind of what we think we already know.

Our desire for the freshness of the new and the trick of the mind to keep us in the story of the past is often the cause of deep sadness and frustration, leading to affairs and sexually compulsive behaviour, and rarely has anything to do with a problem in the relationship itself. Thinking and sex are as incompatible as oil and water. Fantasy, like role play, is not of the mind but is creative and spontaneous; so the real route to bringing back the love in our love life is by getting out of our heads and back to our senses where everything is forever new.

We adults think far too much. I've sat in the treatment room and listened to people telling me that they've heard that mobile telephone signals will go through their bed springs and stop them conceiving, so they've decided to have a bed made with no springs. Someone else told me that she wouldn't let her husband wear brown because it deadens your energy and she'd bought him a magnetic bracelet to boost his sperm. I've had clients who have studied so much that they could go head to head with Sir Robert Winston on *Mastermind* about fertility drugs or the benefits of an all-cabbage diet on pre-menopausal women.

However, if I simply ask patients how their love life is, they're shocked and stumped for answers. Suddenly they've run out of theories and graphs. When I suggest that a couple overhaul their sex life with perhaps a romantic weekend away, some role play, maybe some toys, or really anything that gets them in the mood, they're even more shocked. They protest that they're too busy and tired for that, but if they're too tired to have sex I have no idea how they'll cope with a baby. They blame their in-laws – they come to stay too often – or themselves – "It's my fault, I don't always feel like it" – anything to push away that awkward challenge. When men have erectile problems, the process gets pathologised and there's a prescription for Viagra: it becomes a condition to be medicated, not a temporary blip in a grand passion.

People would rather open up their folders and bring out their charts and tell me all the homework they're putting in – special diets, charted ovulation, correct positions – than go away, rethink and have a heady holiday of sex for the sake of sex. I hear all about cervical mucus quality or the number of sperm in each ejaculation, but to mention the bedroom gets them bristling – in the wrong way. Perhaps if I came out with the statistic that if they had more spontaneous sex more often they would increase their chances of conception by 60 per cent, they would do it. It is very odd to sit with couples who intend to be together for the rest of their lives and raise a family, and watch them make excuses for not making love or finding real sexual expression.

Having sex is just a grown-up version of playing, and the child inside us misses the games. Unlike the dead memories we sometimes evoke during intercourse, games are fresh and alive. Sex is meant to be playful and joyful and provide an arena for fun, experimentation, fantasy, intimacy and loving expression.

If you're lucky, there's a feeling that you get sometimes when making love with someone you are completely passionate about. You feel so joined to him that you almost become him; your body is so open and receptive that it feels as if your womb is unlocking and taking him to your darkest, most primal secret places. I would say this is the prime conception shag! And if you add a bit of desperation into the mix, it can get even more heady. SALLY

The self-consciousness that comes with age and

ageing can extinguish the flame of passion and many couples that I have worked with, non-verbal agreements are made to take the easier option of a cosy cuddle and a peck on the cheek at night.

Good physiological reasons have been found in conventional scientific research for concentrating on the quality of your sex life instead of your ovulation schedule. One study in Australia found that the more frequently men ejaculated, the higher their sperm quality. For years IVF clinics told men that they would raise their sperm count through abstinence, but the researchers discovered that although this resulted in more sperm, much of this multitude was made up of a backlog of old or even damaged sperm which was not improved by being kept stewing! On the other hand, the men who ejaculated on a regular basis had a smaller, but far healthier population of fresh swimmers.

In any case, sperm quality can vary hugely from week to week or even from day to day, as I will explain in more detail later. This variation is another reason why we recommend that people trying to have children have sex every other day – it's pointless having sex only a few times a month when the woman is ovulating in the hope that the man's contribution on those particular days will be up to scratch. By ensuring that a fresh ejaculate of sperm enters the woman's body every other day you increase the odds of at least one champion reaching the egg. Sperm can live from a few hours to anything up to five or even seven days inside the female body, so it makes sense to be sexually active at least seven days before the expected ovulation and a further three days after. But procreation is not an exact science. Having regular sex, among other things, sends a clear message to the body and mind of both the male and female that there is a possibility of conception. The human being is intelligent on all levels and understands what is going on and will respond accordingly.

As for women, regular sex actually stimulates ovulation. Women with active love lives release an ovum in 90 per cent of their cycles, compared to women who abstain, whose egg release drops to less than 50 per cent. Nature doesn't squander its resources if there appears to be little chance of the egg being fertilised!

Not every woman ovulates at the same stage of her cycle – it depends on her health and state of mind from month to month, so it's often impossible to calculate ahead when sex is most likely to "pay off".

Even Taoist philosophy recognises the significance of regular sexual union, signalling the end of "separation" and taking us back "home". Our instinctive drive to couple up, build sexual chemistry and climax is not simply to produce new life, but to reconnect with something far more exciting than anything our body or mind could generate or conjure up. Symbolically, the merging of heaven and earth and the end of separation is expressed through the sexual union of the predominantly male (heaven) and the predominantly female (earth) – where two become one.

Practising acupuncture in the Taoist tradition, and witnessing the success stories of many patients who have resurrected their sex lives and gone on to conceive, I have no doubt that the magic of conscious, connected sex improves your chances of conceiving enormously. Male and female, yin and yang, merge, and the resulting physical, mental and spiritual union nourishes every part of us and reminds us of both our humanity and our spirituality – our sexuality.

Conception is still a mystery as is evident in the low success rates of IVF. It is by no means a guarantee of anything, but in my view human passion and the feeling of being alive cannot be ignored when looking at conception. We are not inert machines performing dry functions trapped in time and space. We are vibrant, dynamic beings with a limitless energy source if we only knew how to harness it. Do you remember how much energy you had when you fell in love, or found a passion for a new project? Where did that come from? This life-giving energy is available to us at all times and one of the most fun and exciting ways to access it is through sexual expression. Being sexual and loving is very human and adds an extra dimension to our life that brings energy and light to everything we do.

The Importance of Orgasms

Did you know that if a woman has an orgasm either a minute before or up to three minutes after her partner, her body will hold on to ten million more sperm than if she came long before or after him or hasn't climaxed at all?

The actual mechanism of the female orgasm is so intricate and influential that new things about it are being discovered every year. Why else would women be able to orgasm if it served no purpose other than pleasure? Pleasure is only one side effect of the sequence of events set in motion by a climax; the rest could make the critical difference between conceiving and not conceiving if a couple are having difficulties. There's even a chance that ovulation can be triggered by surges of hormones pre- or post-orgasm, or, more incredibly still, that the contractions of the uterus in climax might shake the follicles into erupting. Orgasms also have a bearing on how the woman's body treats the sperm that's ejaculated.

The vagina is naturally acidic and hostile to sperm, even containing roving phagocyte cells that will consume invaders – all part of the vagina's self-protection system. Most sperm perishes there and then, although the vagina's pH level is briefly raised so they can survive a short time. If sperm is lucky, it finds a way into the safe haven of the cervical mucus, which has reached lower down the vagina with the cervix, which also dips down as the woman is stimulated. The contractions of the vagina and womb create higher pressure in both. When the woman climaxes, the pressure in the uterus drops sharply, and the cervical mucus and the sperm are effectively sucked up through the cervix and drawn closer to their ultimate destination: the ovum in the fallopian tubes. Also it is worth noting that there is a greater volume of sperm is ejaculated in the male orgasm when the period of arousal is extended. Taking time to stimulate each other will increase the power and potency of the orgasm as a whole. In short, there are good physiological reasons why conception is more likely to happen when you're highly sexually aroused, unthinking and surrendered. Again and again patients have confided that they got pregnant that time they had amazing sex on holiday, or went on top for the first time. There's a real excitement and dynamism, as in Sally's "prime conception shag".

I've had male patients who had given up their old partying lifestyles to go to the gym and sit home with decaf coffee, and I've told them just to go out with the boys and have fun. No, you can't conceive if you're overdoing the party lifestyle, but to exclude that abandon and fun and flirtation from your life altogether is too extreme. Often people are simply bored and worse still, scared, convinced that if they get smashed on tequila they risk having damaged babies with this or that abnormality. The most extreme example I ever witnessed was a woman who had been unable to conceive for years despite her partner having no fertility problems, but who got pregnant as the result of an impromptu wild sexual encounter; freed from all her anxieties and issues by a quantity of champagne, she slept with two men and now has a gorgeous daughter to show for that extraordinary evening. I'm not recommending orgies for everyone, but there must have been sparks flying that night!

One pair of couples I know in the USA had no problem conceiving twice even though they are two gay men and two gay women. Each couple made love in their own rooms, and then the sperm that the men had gathered was passed over to the women (who both happened to be doctors), to be inserted after their own orgasms. Their children were born out of making love and of an orgasm that was fuelled by love, even if the biological mothers and fathers were in separate rooms at the time. When I talk about what is natural, it doesn't have to mean a single heterosexual couple coming together: the important thing is that the energy is generated from love and passion.

I do also believe that a sexy, passionate session can improve your chances of a successful implantation if you have undergone IVF or ICSI or a similar, clinic-based procedure. I suggest to patients who are about to have an "embryo transfer" that they have sex before they go for their appointment, because the heat and chemical reactions of orgasm prime the womb to receive a new inhabitant. Otherwise the new cells are simply transferred from a cold, sterile laboratory environment to a relatively inert uterus, instead of a post-orgasmic one that's pulsing with blood and receptive. I also suggest to people undergoing assisted fertility treatment that they maintain their sex life throughout the whole process leading up to embryo transfer; even though technically it is not needed, I am guessing that those who manage to have regular sex have a higher chance of success than those who are solely focused on their blood results.

A certain erotic dynamism can change your whole body make-up, turning you into a more vibrant, sexual being. When you flirt with others – even with no consequences – your body responds. Look at teenagers, they get excited about going out to socialise, to meet people and make an impression. It may look as if they're spending hours on their wardrobe choices, but in fact it's all part of their honest excitement. When couples find one another and settle down in their nice, comfortable house, they often take this to mean that they can retire from the social scene to some extent, and that lack of interaction makes them less sexual beings overall.

I am very aware that frequent sex isn't practicable for everyone. You can choose to go to the gym or take a walk each day, but you can't compel your partner to have sex with you. In those cases, there's possibly another underlying problem with the relationship, or one or both partners is being dragged down by emotional baggage – I will talk more about this later. I find that when two people are feeling better in their skin and healthier inside and out, the knock-on effect tends to be that they feel sexier and more attractive. They're more excited, they have more energy, and that spills over into an increased libido and a natural spontaneous desire to make love.

Love, sex, relationships and orgasms are all essentially the same thing – they just manifest in many different ways. The starting point is always love, the juice of life, and in many spiritual traditions love is considered the only thing that is real and lasting – everything else comes and goes.

A Balanced Mind

The ancient Chinese teach us that spirit is perfect and always present; it doesn't need resurrecting and it doesn't go anywhere. It's we that come and go, but sometimes it feels like our spirit has been completely buried by everything that has gone on in our lives. By the time we hit our mid-thirties we're mentally a composite of many influences – from our DNA to our parents' relationship, our peers at school, messages in the media and our life experiences. As we grow and respond to the world around us we develop an idea of who we are and what we believe to be true. This construct gives us a personal viewpoint and a framework according to which we live our lives, but if we are not open to reviewing these ideas and actions they can become a trap and restrict our movement through life. They're like bad mental habits that we don't even realise are holding us back.

Over years of practice I've learnt that most of what people tell you in a consultation isn't the full truth. It's not that they intentionally lie, but the past is a story that can be changed in the present and frequently is, as we all need to find reasons for things we don't understand. If you treat patients according to what they tell you, you have to trust that they're right, but usually they are telling you nothing more than stories. Patients tell me that their terrible backache is because they fell out of a tree 35 years ago, or that they can't sleep because their house is on a ley line, or that their terrible indigestion is just like their mother's or their aunt's. Of course, some of these things will be true, but there's normally something more going on when people seek to line themselves up with their parents or anyone else to explain their traits, or worse still, come up with theories based on hearsay. We take things from our experiences and turn them into a story we tell about ourselves; we say we are impatient because our mother always made us wait for treats, or that we have a bad stomach because that's just how it is for all the men in our family. We think we're night owls because we can't sleep, or we have bad blood sugar and that's why we need to binge occasionally. We reckon that we love the adrenaline of stress, or that we're just one of those people who get sluggish and hibernate in winter.

I often ask patients how they feel right now, rather than invite them to recollect their past history, and if, as so often, the answer is "exhausted" or "depressed" or "stuck", my next question is why they don't change what they're doing and so change how they feel.

Recently I saw a new patient who was 39 and had been trying to get pregnant for over five years. Our first meeting was at 7.30am, and as I greeted her in the waiting room with a customary "Good morning", she leapt to her feet, grasped my outstretched hand with both of hers and said, "How are you?"

This very first meeting with a new patient provides invaluable information about how the person operates in the outside world. Sandra had come to me that morning for help but within seconds of meeting her I saw that her knee jerk response to meeting me, and possibly anyone new, was to immediately take on the role of carer and giver.

As Sandra told me about her life, my suspicions were confirmed. She saw herself as the hub of her home (husband and three dogs), her extended family, friends and work colleagues, giving me detailed examples of how she worries about them and is needed in so many ways – and in the same breath highlighting how she feels neglected and unappreciated. I naturally asked her why she took on this role if it was affecting her negatively – and was, possibly, undermining her ability to conceive. But this had never occurred to her and she quickly brushed my questions aside, apparently incapable of seeing how she could change without the risk of the whole group dynamic falling apart. "They need me," she told me defiantly.

When people like Sandra present themselves a certain way – in her case as the worrier and the carer – they have gone far beyond seeing their behaviour and all the associated feelings as an imbalance or something inappropriate. They define it as their personality. Of course, having one of the Five Elements as their causative factor will produce a tendency to one emotional direction, but I've also seen that temporary swing off the scale corrected by a combination of acupuncture and self-willed change in a patient so quickly that it belies the idea that it was ever an ingrained part of who they really are.

Another patient, Julian, was an actor and the son of a well-known artist. He'd been in therapy for years without making any progress, and had a diagnosis of depression, although he came to me for help with his fertility because he and his wife wanted to start a family and he'd been told that he had a very low sperm count. As I walked round the treatment table to take his pulses, his eyes followed my every step. It struck me that the atmosphere in the room was not one of depression – a dragging, sunken greyness – but instead of high tension and anxiety. He could only articulate it as "a black feeling".

Fear is often not given its due. People talk and write articles about depression and the devastating effect it can have, but how many men can admit to feeling afraid, let alone take time off work for anxiety? It is not recognised as something that could be so chronic as to be an illness, and yet I see it cripple people over and again. When Julian described his working week, it was clear that what drove him was a wild surplus of adrenaline and anxiety, and not soul-sapping depression.

After he had had treatment over several weeks he started to show results. One day, he turned up for his appointment and said in surprise that he'd noticed a difference since the last treatment; this time he actually called it "an absence of fear". He seemed refreshed and less manic, and said he'd drunk less alcohol than usual because he hadn't needed to cope with "the black feeling". At the next consultation, he had swung back into extreme anxiety but this time he recognised it for what it was, simply a passing feeling. I continued treating him and gradually that swing back to "normal" stabilised. He found it easier to work and he was able to father a child.

He eventually told me his earliest memory of that black feeling. When he was a child his father would force him into his study and sit him down at his side. The boy would be given paper and a pen and told to do his homework while his father worked. It imbued him with a terrible feeling that, as a seven-year-old he couldn't place. It grew worse when his father would ask him to hand over the pieces of paper and let him read the story or essay he'd written. No wonder as an adult he couldn't bear to tie himself to a desk all day.

No one exists in a fixed state. You don't need to remain scared for ever because of a childhood experience. Many of my patients describe aspects of their lives that sound absolutely miserable and yet they battle on as though they cannot possibly escape their situation. They have lost a sense of perspective. They hate their job but feel unable to change it. They don't like where they live but they'll come out with a reel of reasons for staying there. Julian thought he had to drink to work and almost saddled himself with a serious alcohol problem in the process, without seeking out the source of the emotion that drove him to be so scared and restless.

Many years ago I treated a woman called Charlotte who was 32 and had been doing everything possible to conceive for almost three years. There was nothing wrong with her medically and she said she'd had a happy, stable upbringing and continued to enjoy her adult life. She called her life "picture-book perfect". She and her husband had been very successful in business and she felt secure and loved by him. The only thing missing was a baby.

Not long after starting treatment her father was diagnosed with lung cancer and told he had three months to live. He also told Charlotte that he had excluded her from his will because he thought she was financially stable and well off through her own endeavours, and wouldn't need further support from him. Her brother had very little money and was assured a significant figure by their father, and her sister would get the balance. They were all a little mortified by their father's announcement, and had promised Charlotte that after his death they would share out the inheritance equally, but the damage was done. Charlotte felt rejected – as though her own father thought she was worthless.

She felt that her idyllic life had fallen apart overnight, and she sank into a very dark place full of self-loathing and fear. I worked with her to support her through this sudden depression and early grief, and she did her best to understand why her father's announcement had been such a blow. This involved taking a close look at the story she'd told herself about both her upbringing and her current life.

When she was little, her father was a god. She was devoted to him, and described the moment when he walked in the door in the evening as "like the sun coming out from behind a cloud". Her father was devoted to her too, and would take her everywhere with him, but one afternoon when she was twelve, he took her out with him and introduced her to a female friend he called Jane. The three of them spent the day together but Charlotte felt very uncomfortable with this woman, and noticed, even though she was young, how close her father seemed to her. She never did find out if her father was having an affair with Jane but from then on she felt that the special relationship she'd had with her father changed irrevocably.

When her father told her about the will, she was pitched back to this time when she'd seen him through different eyes and been disappointed in him, and left feeling alone. She hadn't realised at twelve how deeply she'd been hurt, or that she'd felt betrayed. Rather than talk about her feelings with anyone, she'd tried to cut her father out of her affections without thinking. That emotional separation marked her. From that day on she'd gradually come to see everything as her responsibility, and felt driven to create and control a perfect life that couldn't be shaken by someone else's betrayal. The woman I met at the first consultation was strong, charismatic and determined to maintain and defend this life, and her father had obviously understood that she needed nothing from him. He in turn had felt rejected, although at a conscious level all he had seen was success and independence. His last will and testament reflected this unspoken dynamic.

When she stepped back and examined this chain of events, Charlotte saw the pattern of emotions underlying them. She managed to talk to her father and found herself ready to forgive him. She shifted gears in her own life too – she began to enjoy the comfortable life she had created for herself without striving to defend it or submit it to anyone's approval.

Her father defied his diagnosis and lived a full year. Charlotte was with him the night before he died and felt no resentment or anger, only love. She conceived her first child exactly three months later to the night.

Another client, Robert, had been told that he had an incredibly low sperm count – just 40 or 50 in a sample. He was only 29 and newly in love with an incredibly sweet woman with whom he wanted to have children. They hadn't been trying long before they went for tests, only to be brought up short by this dire result.

When I put my hand on his chest to check his temperature, I was struck by how fragile he was. It was as if his whole body was going to suck me down and keep me there. Physical contact, any form of contact, was obviously a deep need for him – even with this tremendously kind, affectionate girlfriend right there with him, he was still desperate for any affection. It was as though he couldn't produce this feeling for himself and so needed to absorb that care from others.

He also wanted to help others, and told me his plans for learning to be a hypnotherapist and putting together a package of ways to assist people to lose weight. He'd done all his research and knew there was a good market out there, but you could see what it really meant to him – an opportunity to care for others.

I asked about his medical history and he told me that as a nineteen-year-old he had been recruited by a fast-growing technology company that prized his brains and put him on to a fast track for promotion. He was full of ideas and fresh perspectives on the business, and his bosses began to portray him as the company superstar who was destined for great things. He worked hard, pushing himself to meet their expectations, but at 21 he was completely burnt out and suffered a nervous breakdown.

He collapsed and left work, battling depression and paranoia at home. He was given antidepressants and counselling, and managed to get disability benefits. He was out of the workplace for years, living in much reduced circumstances. The psychosomatic symptoms that he suffered could be crippling. He felt dizzy constantly, and his stomach lining was gnawed by ulcers. Slowly he came back to a state where he could function and return to work, but it was clear that this recovery had been only partial.

He would, he told me, worry about the smallest thing. If he needed to go to the shops for groceries, he'd worry that maybe he wouldn't have enough money to pay for them, or that, worse still, he'd get to the till and find he'd left his wallet at home. Or what if he made his purchase successfully but dropped the receipt on the way out of the store, and was apprehended for shoplifting, unable to prove his innocence? Much of this inner dialogue never reached the open air, and those around him would have been surprised to know how consumed he was.

He would have enthusiasm for new projects like re-fitting the kitchen, but when confronted with all the boxes of flat-pack cabinets and furniture, he would end up in a foetal position on the sofa, unable to believe he could cope. The problem was not that he couldn't do these things, but that the extreme panic induced by the mere thought of them would whirl him into a fear that was deep, dark and entirely out of proportion.

As this story came tumbling out of him, I realised that it hadn't even occurred to him that this level of ongoing stress could in any way be connected to his low sperm count.

After the first few sessions where he talked and started to make connections, he told me that he felt filled out from the inside for once, not just hollow. And he also talked about the first time he had experienced the intense anxiety. When he was seven, his father had left him and his mother and two sisters, and as a little boy, he had felt a huge burden as the new "man" of the house. He felt his mother expected too much of him, and he took on responsibility for everyone in the home being well and happy. That precocious responsibility was probably the reason his employers at the tech company snapped him up, but it was also just a well-developed cover for the seven-year-old boy who needed comfort and reassurance. When that cover began to crack, he broke down.

After a year of regular treatment and support, and a significant improvement in his general well-being, his sperm count had bounded up, and he and his girlfriend conceived their first child.

Sometimes people will, out of habit, create brand-new burdens for themselves, seemingly as a distraction from their current problems. Finding the root cause of someone's suffering is not an easy process. What I do try to do is instil in them the discipline to stop their mind from drifting back into their "story" and making fear or regret their default setting.

It is an uncomfortable truth that we humans create and can carry around a lot of guilt, fear and other negative emotions. Heartache seems to be part of our natural make-up, and even if there's nothing present in our day-to-day life to make us suffer, we will go out and find it. We get used to the dark and say we're "fine" when we're carrying around a heavy load of emotional baggage, which stops us being who we really are and living our lives to the full.

Being in the Moment

So often our personal story with its load of unresolved psychological baggage and an inability to "be in the moment" are intertwined. We define who we are by our story. It's impossible to root yourself in the present when you're drunk with thoughts and emotions from the past or longing for something in the future. By getting rid of old problems and curbing your fantasies, you sober up and free yourself to be in the present moment and be your Self, as you really are.

Acupuncture, at a very basic physical level, can foster this kind of awareness via the insertion of a needle into an acupuncture point, which focuses your attention right there – right now. This momentary intervention, which immediately affects and balances the flow of energy, has a spontaneous homeostatic knock-on effect throughout the body, mind and spirit. This tangible response to treatment is echoed in many of the case studies portrayed in this book: each experience is unique, but it shows how everyone can access their true self regardless of their current problems or difficulties.

Taoist philosophy tells us that our natural and permanent state is one of contentment and peace, and that this is indestructible. This peace lies at the core of everything and is the essence of humanity. Some people call this the "God within", but whatever name you want to give it, the important thing to remember is that it is not something you have to find or create; it exists at the heart of all of us. The challenge for you is to raise this consciousness from under the layers of your stories and the illusory "self" created by your thoughts and feelings.

I often try to teach patients about this when I see them worrying and fretting about all kinds of things. They look at me as if I am mad and then give me more reasons why they feel so terrible. They're married to misery. That is not to say there are no real problems in life; it's just these problems are ultimately ephemeral, they are impermanent, part of life's ebb and flow – just as in the natural world there are disasters, but the root of existence is one of stillness, peace and love.

So how do we connect with this blissful state? Turn your back on what you see as your problematic life and pay attention to what truly exists within you. It is an act of faith. We talk about "my life" or "my problems" as if they were our possessions – things that we carry on our backs and make us feel like somebody and oh-so-very important. We take what happens around us far too seriously and, worse still, find our identity through them. Most of the time we believe in the struggle that our mind and ego would have us believe is the only way.

Being in the moment or coming to your senses, means exactly that – fully feeling and experiencing what is going on at the moment. For example, if you stop thinking for a second you will be aware of the chair beneath your legs, the smells in the room and the colours around you. Being consciously present as we live each moment of our lives is grounding and reassuring, and connects us with the "blissful state" – whereas too much thinking and too much agonising can take us off to imaginary places that destabilise us and distract us from the reality of the moment.

If Only…

"If only we had started trying for a baby five years ago." "If only I had not had that termination, my child would now be fifteen." "If only I had played tennis and not rugby and not got kicked in the – you know where." "If only I had started IVF earlier." "If only I had heard about you earlier." "If only we had enough money for egg donation." "If only he would stop smoking…"

In our culture playing the "if only" game, much like engaging in gossip, can feel compelling and attractive, but in truth it is something we do to avoid living in the present moment. "If only" takes us backwards and forwards, visiting the past that has gone and the future that doesn't exist, but actually serves no purpose. It just gives us a faux "experience" which brings more pain and prevents us from being true to ourselves.

My patient Marcie not only played the "if only" game with flair, but was a genius at knowing when to play the "if only" trump card that could flatten any optimism I offered in the here and now.

Marcie was 42 years old and had met her partner Simon a year earlier. Simon had been coming to me for treatment for years and was in great shape. He (now in his late fifties) was delighted to have met Marcie and truly excited that they had both agreed they wanted to start a family.

Marcie came to me reluctantly – and in confidence

told me, "It's not going to work, you know. My hormone levels are all over the place and have never been right since I started my menstrual cycle."

Without drawing breath she continued, "You see, there's a problem with implantation because of a termination I had in my thirties. That coupled with my crazy hormones – it doesn't look very hopeful." She paused. "If only I had met Simon after my menopause rather than now. He thinks there's still a chance of us having children. I know I'm going to disappoint him and he'll want to move on – I'm sure."

This disclosure of her history, her view on her current state and her fears of abandonment were delivered with such conviction it was hard to challenge her in any way.

Marcie and Simon were clearly deeply in love. They spoke of each other with sweetness and affection but it was obvious that Simon's excitement around the possibility of becoming a father juxtaposed with Marcie's fear of letting him down was dampening the their newfound love. Most importantly, their sex life was now being compromised by Marcie's reluctance to find time for regular sex as she feared this would only serve to set Simon up for disappointment.

"If only we had met in our twenties," Marcie lamented on her second visit to me, staring out of the window and lost in thought. "I am sure we would have had lots of children had we started back then."

This was Marcie's preferred position, loss of what

could have been, and fear of what she undoubtedly believed would happen. Lamenting the past and fearing the future was familiar to her and this became apparent as I learnt about other areas of her life.

"I think if my mother had been more available to me as a child I would have found some direction in my work, but I've just floated from one thing to another so it is very unlikely, now at 42, I am going to find the big career." Every sentence that came from her was conveyed with confidence and charm and any attempt to challenge her belief that she was trapped by the story of her past was met with a "You don't seem to understand…" glare, followed by a "…but never mind" smile, and then straight back to the accounts of what should and could have been.

From a medical point of view there was nothing wrong with Marcie. On paper her hormone levels were normal for her age and after only one year of having unprotected sex with Simon not being pregnant was well within the range of "normal" by most fertility experts' standards.

"I have little doubt you can get pregnant Marcie," I boldly said one day, trying to direct her away from her negative memories and fears. "Providing you are having sex every other day throughout your cycle and looking after yourself – I'd be surprised if it doesn't happen in the next year."

My confidence and directness seemed to get through

and for a second she was lost for words. "Really?" she said and turned to look out of the window. Realising I was about to lose her again, I went all out. "In fact – based on my three decades of experience I would wager that if you committed to having sex every other day for the next six months and be *totally present* to each and every act – you'll be pregnant."

"You're on!" she shot back. "I love a wager." I won the bet. Three months later Marcie was pregnant. There is nothing mysterious or surprising about this story – just as for many other things in life, we have to be present to each and every moment as one creates the next. Disappearing into regret, fantasy, memory or any other mental state, distracts us from the reality of the now.

Conception happens in the here and now. It is an event that mirrors orgasm, when everything appears to stop for an imperceptible moment, rendering us able only to feel and not think, as we are reminded of what it is like to be truly present. Marcie came back into the here and now with the prospect of a task that involves not only the mental, but more importantly the physical – the physical act of making love and being present to the one you love.

Faith

What is meant by faith? The confident belief in the

truth? Some kind of religious following? In this context it is the willingness to give up control, but that doesn't mean doing nothing and nor does it mean relinquishing control to anyone else. In my experience, most people who have "failed" to conceive feel that they have no other option than to take control and do something about the situation. This at first brings a temporary sense of relief, but very soon, as each new strategy fails, desperation and fear dominate the picture. This of course further exacerbates the problem. It's like being in a maze with no way out.

Whether we accept it or not, we all have that capacity to have faith. Some believe in the power of their vitamin pills, their own intellect, the skill of their doctor or the magic of the acupuncture needles; some in God. Faith is part of being human and it is not prescriptive, but its essence is rooted deep within us.

When things go wrong, like finding out you can't get pregnant, this perceived wrongness compounds our illusion of separateness and the sense that we have to work it all out for ourselves. "If we can just keep control we will be OK," we think. Our doubts, cynicism and fear of anything greater than us is a natural reaction, but it is ultimately just a construct of our mind, the voice of the self-made ego that will tell us anything to survive.

If you ask any human being what they ultimately want, you always end up with the same answer: to be happy. To live spontaneously and let go of the idea that we are somehow in control of achieving happiness takes a great leap of faith. We are conditioned to believe that "happiness" is out there somewhere; to be found in a car or a job or a child. In our bid to maintain this illusion of control, rather than find the happiness that already exists within us, we find temporary comfort by constructing our own confident belief in what we see as the truth and then find others who will collude with our story to strengthen our case. This rather clumsy and exhausting strategy to achieve happiness and the things we believe we need is rife in our culture and now even extends to making babies. Juliet described her situation like this:

I'd had my first son when I was 34 and my second at 36, and both times my husband and I conceived almost at the first attempt. It never crossed my mind that I might have problems with my fertility, but I had been interested to read a series of features in a women's magazine about Gerad and the stories of women who'd been to his clinic. Each article seemed to encourage a wave of new people willing to try acupuncture, and then a new article covering the successful treatments.

Acupuncture wasn't something I'd considered myself, partly because I didn't think it fitted with my faith as a Christian – I just thought it was a bit hocus-pocus.

About a year later I was in a different position. My husband had wanted to try for a third child, but we hadn't had the same luck. I had had a major health scare and was told by my doctors to avoid pregnancy for a while, but when I was given the all-clear my head just felt messed up. I wasn't sure if I really wanted a third child in case it affected my career badly, and I'd have to rejig my life entirely.

I had some therapy, which helped, but one day I decided to go and talk to Gerad, because I felt something was wrong with my fertility system. I was a bit nervous about going, and I remember walking into the treatment room and there were all these Buddhas everywhere and thinking, "God, do you want me to do this?" In the end I said a brief prayer and said, "God, I give this session to you." I actually ended up talking a lot about faith with Gerad. He's a trained psychotherapist so he's very easy to talk to, and the first few sessions felt just like chat therapy. The needles didn't do anything in particular until the fourth visit, when he put one point in and it just felt like a pane of glass fell away.

It was as though I'd been wearing these glasses that had told me, "You've had a really successful career, why are you trying for a baby?" and now suddenly my body took over and said, "You're mad! Why are you compromising your fertility by thinking about your career when you really do want a baby?" I discovered that it really did matter to me that I had another child. The next month I was shocked and delighted to find that I was pregnant.

I think the connection between mind and body in conception is absolutely fascinating. I know that acupuncture made a huge difference to me, and I don't think it's "magic". For me it's been quite a spiritual thing. It's not like prayer, where you're talking directly to God, but it does give you a sort of stillness in yourself, and that brings you back in line with your faith. I saw Gerad the week before I conceived and I remember going into the session feeling very angry with God, and being embarrassed because I didn't know why I felt that way. I came out feeling very humble and couldn't believe I'd been so worked up before.

We live in a world of laptops and wifi and we're so full on, and rather than being swept away by that raging torrent of city life where you're bringing up your children and juggling work, the needles seem to restore that peace in your soul where you connect to God.

Stop Trying

Everyone has heard the example of the couple trying for a baby for years and years before finally deciding to adopt; and then, within months of happily settling into new parenthood, a natural pregnancy occurs. I have heard this story recounted so many times by patients who are hoping for a family, and yet when I suggest they think about how this example might help them to look at conception from a different point of view, they tend to take me at face value – assuming that I am suggesting that they, too, go straight for adoption.

Every day in my practice I hear people who have been diagnosed with unexplained infertility telling me how long they have been "trying" to get pregnant. Trying to do anything takes effort and often the exhausted look on people's faces as they recount the numerous cycles of conception attempts tells a weary tale. Here is our dilemma.

We used to use the term "to fall pregnant" because we recognised that it was an involuntary act. We cannot *think* our way into conceiving just as we cannot think ourselves into falling in love.

We're told time and time again that if we want something we have to knuckle down and fight for it, to organise and rally our resources and push ourselves to our limits to chase that reward. It is absolutely true of many things achieved in life, but it doesn't mean it is the best way to do it. The things that are truly magic in life are the things we have no control over: falling asleep, falling in love, falling pregnant. Three absolutely basic things that in their absence can derail you completely, while seeming ludicrously easy for others.

These three fundamental realities of life happen when we are not trying because they are rooted in the part of us that has no conscious choice. There is a part of humanity that must submit to the will of nature and accept that something deep inside us has the ultimate say. The ancient Chinese recognised that, just as they held no sway over the movement of the Earth and the perceived rising and the setting of the sun, they had no control of their waking and sleeping, and so they surrendered to natural forces and accepted their place as part of their pattern and design. This extended to their understanding of fertility, which was in turn built on their knowledge of nature, where some years the seeds would grow and flourish, producing a strong harvest, while other years they would struggle to survive.

In the West we've been conditioned to think we're in control; we'll persuade ourselves into a relationship with a partner who never really "clicked" with us, we'll nod off with sleeping pills, and we'll conceive on target just when we want to. But, for all our medical innovations, I see couples who have experienced problems with conceiving time and again, only to conceive just when they had given up hope and relaxed.

Wanting something can be dangerous. By that I don't mean that it's wrong to want a particular thing, or that you should think that you don't deserve something, but that the act of yearning and obsessing over it can create a tension that is counterproductive to the very goal you're trying to achieve.

The idea of stopping trying is terrifying to people. They have been trying to have a child for so long with such diligence and focus that they think that longed-for pregnancy is just around the corner. It's like someone who has always chosen the same lottery numbers, and won't change them in case next week is the one when they come up.

To stop trying suggests the end of the road, and all options exhausted, but it's more like a respite. This shift of focus is often the beginning of a shift in energy that allows something in you finally to move and change after years of being held back by your own earnest, commendable but often exhausting efforts.

Falling pregnant is about trusting and believing it could happen; we need to get out of the way so that the potent forces of nature can move through us and do what is needed. Charlotte says:

We weren't trying to have our oldest son, Thomas. I knew I had endometriosis as it had been diagnosed six months before Tim and I got married. We'd been told that conception might be a problem but at that point I wasn't fussed about having children and it didn't really bother either of us whether we had kids or not.

I struggled to get my head round it when I first found out I was pregnant. My life would have gone down a very different path if I hadn't had Thomas. I was working in the fashion business and for want of a better word I was a cold-hearted workaholic bitch! I was motivated by money, fast cars and nice holidays. Looking back now, I suppose I wasn't a very nice person. Having him triggered the maternal instinct, and it softened me around the edges. It was like having a carrot dangled in front of you; I thought, "If this is what it's like having a boy, imagine what it would be like to have a girl too!"

When Thomas was a couple of years old we started trying for a second child, without thinking it would be difficult, but we had no luck. My first reaction was anger and frustration. There was very little out there for couples going through secondary infertility and I found that a lot of people were unsympathetic. Even my own mother couldn't see why we were so set on having another child; she thought we should be happy with what we had. I can remember walking around the supermarket and seeing mums screaming at their five children with filthy clothes and running noses and thinking, "This is unfair!" I was so angry that I almost felt like running over and physically hurting them.

It was really odd dealing with those extreme feelings because the only time I'd felt emotions like that was from a business perspective in the cut-throat world of work. A friend was going through fertility treatments for a first child at the same time as me, and she was treated very sympathetically. It seemed that we were just supposed to deal with it.

The drug I was taking, Clomid, makes you feel like you're living with the worst PMT in the world, permanently. I imagine it made me very difficult to live with. Physically it was dreadful, but mentally I felt at least I was doing something, so every time I got off the hormonal rollercoaster I just wanted to get right back on it again.

After several unsuccessful rounds of IUI with Clomid, they switched me to gonadotropin drugs, and that's when the fun starts, because you start having the injections and I can remember that feeling of my ovaries throbbing 24/7 and horrible bloating where you can't get your clothes done up any more. We had IUI, where the sperm is gathered and then injected directly into your womb at ovulation, and after they'd put the sperm in, there was cramping because my uterus was aggravated. I think we had nine or ten rounds of IUI altogether. On the sixth or seventh I got to day 90 after insemination without having a period but although I had pregnancy symptoms, my tests came back negative.

My GP was concerned because there was a slim chance that I had conceived, but that the embryo was developing ectopically. When I went for a scan it revealed instead that I had polycystic ovary syndrome, and that was why I hadn't had a period for so long. The consultant I saw suggested ovarian drilling, in which the surgeon makes between five and ten holes in the ovary; a process that is supposed to regulate your cycle, although no one knows how it works.

I remember walking down to the operating theatre not thinking anything of having holes drilled in my ovaries. I didn't question anything because I always felt like I was being proactive and that if I did enough procedures we'd find the right one and I would conceive.

I used to use fertility support group message boards on the internet and although they were really helpful, they also made me impatient because you could see women who'd had the same treatments at the same time and even at the same clinic as you and were producing more eggs, or better-quality eggs that could be frozen. My eggs were never good enough for freezing, and people who were able to freeze their embryos didn't have to go through as many doses of fertility drugs.

I measured everything in life in the cost of a night's worth of fertility drugs, at £200 a time. We had several tipping points financially when my husband, Tim, would say, "Charlotte, we really can't borrow any more money." We stopped having holidays, we stopped going out, and we started rationing what we bought at the supermarket. I'd always been used to buying nice clothes, having worked in fashion, and suddenly I was getting everything in Tesco. You adapt your whole life around it. You don't realise what it's like until you're halfway through it, and then you can't stop.

The crisis came when I got ovarian hyper-stimulation syndrome and had to be rushed into hospital. I was very, very sick, and was more swollen than I'd been when I was seven months pregnant with Thomas. I can still see my mum next to my hospital bed saying, "Charlotte, you are going to kill yourself and you've got a little boy who needs you. Please, please will you stop all this?"

For me that was a real low mentally and physically, the absolute pits. We were at the end of our tether. We had no money to do any more. I felt wrecked. I'd put on two stone because of all the drugs I'd been taking for years, and I felt I had no marriage left. I knew I was being a bad mother. Poor Thomas was being dragged around to my scans with me. I'd pick him up after school and he'd come to the clinic with me and sit there counting my follicles!

It's a very weird set-up that you find yourself in, and I was almost ready to give up, but I remember begging my husband to let me have one more go. He was reluctant, and I said, "Don't worry, they know about the hyperstimulation now; they'll be really careful and I'll know what to look out for. If I don't do it, I'll go mad."

One of my friends spotted an article on Gerad in *Eve* magazine which was all about a journalist who'd had problems conceiving. Apart from the acupuncture, Gerad had advised her to do what she'd always wanted, which was to buy a cat. Soon after she got the cat, she conceived. We'd been in talks to take part in a documentary by Sir Robert Winston on infertility, and when we had lunch with one of the researchers, I mentioned that I was considering acupuncture and she told me she'd heard good things about Gerad.

As soon as I got home I phoned to make an appointment. I was very sceptical, and Tim was even more so, but I had an idea that it might help with more IUI treatments.

I remember walking into the treatment room at Gerad's clinic, and I don't think I even said hello to him, I just said, "Don't turn round and tell me I need to get a kitten, because I don't really like animals." I can still picture his face, thinking, "Jeez, we've got a right one here."

He often reminds me about that first session, because he says I was all "I want a baby, except I don't want a baby, I want a girl, and she's got to have curly hair and a little nose that's all stuck up at the front here and she's wearing a pink babygrow with a lace collar and I'm not giving up until I've got her!" And he was sitting there thinking, "And you won't!"

He explained that we'd try to get me through one natural cycle without drugs and once I'd had a period, and gotten into my next cycle, I could try IVF if I wanted. I replied that he was lucky I was even giving him one natural cycle, and how he didn't slap me and tell me to go away, I have no idea!

I demanded to know what I needed to do if I didn't need to get a cat, and he just said, "You just need another focus in life, Charlotte." That statement really struck me. Afterwards I walked out of the clinic to the Tube and phoned Tim, and said, "You know, it's really weird." And he said, "What's weird?" "I don't know, but I feel really weird, and do you know? It doesn't really matter if we don't have another baby because everything's going to be all right." I think Tim thought Gerad must have drugged me or something! When we were sitting in the kitchen having dinner that night he said, "Will you talk me through this process?" He thought I'd been hypnotised and I had to reassure him that we'd just talked and I'd had the needles stuck in.

At this stage I think I thought of Gerad as just a nice chap you could pop along and chat to, so it was more like psychotherapy than anything else. I didn't feel anything in particular when the needles were applied.

In the small hours of the morning after my second session I woke up leaking breast milk. My nightie was soaked with it. It was over ten years since Thomas had been born, and I hadn't breastfed him. It was like when you're breast-feeding and haven't expressed any milk for eight hours, and then the baby cries and sets it off. I went to bed feeling completely normal, and woke up at 2am to this. That's when I realised that the acupuncture was having a physical effect. There's no way I can make milk leak from my breasts because of something psychosomatic. It shifted my whole mindset.

A couple of weeks later I was cleaning out the garage and something odd happened. I realised that I was starting my period. Every period I'd had before then had begun with 48 hours of agony because of my endometriosis, so I hadn't guessed that I was about to menstruate. It was my first ever pain-free period, and for me it just compounded what had happened with the milk.

I was ready to start the drugs which would regulate me again, but at the next session with Gerad, when he was checking my pulses, he told me to go home and try a pregnancy test because he thought it had finally happened. I used to buy pregnancy and ovulation tests on the internet in bulk in those days and when you've peed on as many sticks as I had, and never seen the double blue line, it's really strange when you see it. I did three tests in a row, and they all came up positive. I decided they must be wrong because they were cheap, so I rushed out to the supermarket and bought several more, and they all had double blue lines too.

I didn't really believe it till my scan, and my pregnancy was nerve-wracking because I had bleeding throughout. I kept on seeing Gerad and Max was born at 39 weeks, to our delight. Five months after Max was born, I was at Gerad's clinic complaining that my boobs hurt and I felt odd, and that if I didn't know better I'd say I was pregnant, and he checked my pulses and said, "Well, I think you are!" "I can't be!" Well, I was, and that was my little girl, Clementine, so you can imagine that by the time she was born I thought I'd won the lottery.

Five-Element acupuncture has changed my life and not just because I was able to have children after that long journey. It's made me a much better person. It's made me really look at how I am. Six years ago I was angry about life, full stop. I did fight it because I thought I didn't want to change too much of who I was, and he said, "Look, you're always going to be feisty, we're never going to take that away from you, but just learn to channel it." I'd blocked everyone and everything out of my life and become this hugely focused person – well, almost a machine – who ram-raided her way through life. I definitely have more of a cup half full rather than a cup half empty attitude now. I've changed jobs to work with an organisation which arranges international exchanges for students, which uses my old business skills but also gives me a chance to help look after teenagers who are far from home and sometimes quite troubled. It feels worthwhile in a way that my old management career never did. It can be tough with three children, especially when two are just thirteen months apart, but I count my blessings every day.

For someone like Charlotte or Juliet, to let go of control can be an incredibly liberating and powerful experience and can have surprising results. To accept that the struggle may be unhelpful and that you are best served by surrendering to or giving up whatever it is you are fighting for is an act of faith. It is not about losing – far from it – it's just about having the humility to accept your place in the world, trusting that by taking the path of least resistance something will change for the better. Along the way you might discover life-changing things about yourself, as Charlotte did. Charlotte was totally distracted by her new baby when she accidently conceived her longed-for little girl. She certainly wasn't "trying" at that point.

This is where things get tricky. Anything we try to achieve where the decision is made from our head is less likely to work out well. A good decision is not a calculated thought but the outcome of a complex internal process, often unknowable by our conscious mind. We wake in the morning and somehow we know we have to change something; or without even realising it we find ourselves doing something differently. As I mentioned earlier, our minds are wonderful instruments when used correctly but pale into insignificance in the presence of our "true self" when it comes to knowing what is best for us. Being yourself and living in a way that is congruent with who you are and what you love taps into something greater than you could ever imagine. "But I would love a baby," I hear you cry. "Is that not true for me and who I am?" Yes, of course, but now consider leaving that thought alone, enjoy your life as it is today and change what you know you can and leave the rest to work its own way out.

A couple called Andrew and Catherine came to see me. They lived a very safe life; they had jumped through all the right hoops, graduated from the right universities, secured good jobs and bought a flat with a reasonable mortgage so that they could save some money every month.

When I first saw them for treatment, I was struck by the sensation of claustrophobia that rose off them both. It wasn't just that they seemed trapped; they were also resentful and they kept chiming, "disap-pointed". They had been told to be sensible and that this would bring its own reward.

As a practitioner it's my job to stay neutral and not pass judgment on the lives of patients. After all, if I've learnt anything over the years of working with people, it's that every individual and couple is unique and that they need to find their own way of living. Andrew and Catherine's life would have been perfect for plenty of other people but it clearly wasn't right for them. I asked Andrew, "If this is the route of your choice, what does the outcome tell you?" and he simply replied, "It ain't working."

After that we talked about what they could do to change things. I continued treating Andrew and one of my colleagues started seeing Catherine. We didn't make any specific suggestions but hoped that treatment would relieve that sense of claustrophobia. After a while, they made a decisive swerve off the track.

They sold their modest house and took out a whopping mortgage on a new place on the outskirts of London needing a lot of work. They told me with glee that they'd lied to their parents about the extent of the debt they'd taken on, and threw themselves into doing up the house. They'd been wanting to get out of town for a while but had put the move on hold till they had a child. Now, despite the stress of an imprudent mortgage, they began to enjoy themselves. At weekends they were out at flea markets and antique dealers, picking up all kinds of oddities for the house. There was something uncharacteristically extravagant and theatrical about this new joint project. They even asked where my paint supplies for the clinic came from, because they fancied a gold ceiling. They raided their sacrosanct savings fund and took an extravagant holiday because they had no idea why they'd been saving up in the first place. Their lives seemed to flesh out and fill with colour, literally. Where before they'd told me that they'd only ever gone out on Friday and Saturday nights, they now started going out on a Monday or a Wednesday, and staying out late instead of rushing back to bed for an early night. Rather than waking up shattered and hung-over, they were surprised to find they had more energy.

With all these changes, they had stopped focusing on having a child, and when Catherine had a positive pregnancy test it seemed incidental to the rest of their news. It had become the most normal, natural thing in the world.

A Fresh Perspective

Choosing a job, a lifestyle or when to start a family or in fact anything in life, is exactly that: a choice. This for the most part feels conscious and deliberate – but is it? We also make thousands of tiny unconscious choices, made every day of our lives that either resonate with or move further from our own true nature, and every time we choose something in life we are playing out our own story or as the ancient Chinese saw it – fulfilling our destiny. We can see this as a tremendous freedom, but how do we know or make sure those choices and decisions are being made from the right part of our selves?

We put a lot of energy into clinging to choices we have made in our heads, being attached to what we have created and believe to be right. Very often we have invested years of hard work and determination to achieve our goals and we will not give them up lightly even when we know our experience of them is hollow and empty. It is easy to get stuck, or fail to realise how discontented we've become.

Problems with jobs, workmates or family seem insurmountable, but they only are if we let them be so. We need to be flexible in life and open to inevitable change. Even the most organised, according-to-plan existence can be derailed by a great misfortune or a lucky chance. I believe it's as possible to conceive a baby at 40 as at 20 if we're prepared to change and adapt with the passing of time and maintain our physical, mental and spiritual well-being throughout life.

One couple who came to see me, Ann and Scott, thought ahead to plan the lifestyle they wanted. They had started a buy-to-let business because they thought it would give them freedom to enjoy their lives without being chained to a desk or employed by someone. They had been very successful and were now ready to have children, but something was wrong.

Ann wanted to have children as she was in her late thirties and felt she was running out of time. Scott was less rushed. When pushed, in a single session without Ann, he admitted that he wanted to maintain the freedom they'd hoped for when they set up their business. He said he wouldn't try to persuade Ann either way, because she wanted them to get on with having a baby now.

After a little more thought and some shaking up, the two of them decided to take a year off from the baby conveyor belt and hired someone to look after their business for twelve months. They took off for Canada, got hold of a Winnebago and travelled all the way to Chile. Ann hadn't been as keen as Scott but she took the risk and ended up loving the trip. They conceived their first child in Brazil at Mardi Gras.

People often tell me they can't leave a job which makes them miserable. That statement just digs their pit a little deeper. I'm not anti-career, and I definitely don't think that women need to be out of the office and back in the kitchen to conceive, but I am suggesting that there is a balance to be struck between work and life, and that everyone should develop their ability to sound out who they are and what works for them.

I remember watching a friend of mine who was hoping to get pregnant go through a real renaissance after realising that her life in London was intolerable and maybe affecting her fertility. She was 40 at the time, living in a dingy basement flat with a younger boyfriend whom she adored, and teaching an oversize class of demanding children, many of whom came from deprived backgrounds. Worn out and tired, she'd half convinced herself that her boyfriend was bound to leave her for someone else, and no amount of reassurance helped her see how ridiculous that was.

She'd slipped into bulimia, and as friends we were all worried about her because she was getting thinner and thinner.

In the end she didn't sign herself up for therapy, counselling or acupuncture. She took up her boyfriend's suggestion that they move to his home country of Spain and begin a new life. They moved to a tiny village where he got a job in the local tourist industry and she freelanced as an English teacher for local kids. They had time to hike into the mountains every day and Ann, who is a country girl at heart, blossomed. When I visited them I could hardly recognise her as she looked like a different woman. They had no problem conceiving their first child, only three months after relocating.

There's no absolute right or wrong; you have to take action and do things in your own way. That might mean at times being completely inert or manic, it doesn't matter, as long as you are firmly rooted in the part of you that is content and at peace. In the constant flux of life, when you follow your true path, your "pendulum" is able to return to the balancing point, the middle, rather than swing to one polarity or the other, and that's what will keep you safe, well and in the fertile zone (for more on the working of the pendulum, see page 248). When people start to live this way they see all kinds of health benefits. They sleep a little better, enjoy exercising, feel more at peace, have more fun and, while enjoying being who they are, very often finally conceive.

If something is not working then change surely is a solution. The hardest part is working out what needs to change and how to do it. It takes a great deal of courage to take an honest look at ourselves and be prepared to change the things we think are right but know deep down are wrong and are making us sick and unhappy. Real choice does not come from the mind but from the spirit. A choice is something we feel in ourselves, our bodies; our instinctive compass guiding us as our life unfolds. It is only when we start listening to our self and our truth that we can take full responsibility for the choices we make and the life we lead.

Intention

At the beginning of the first meeting with every patient I ask a simple question: "If you could have anything from this treatment, what would you put at the top of your list?" Very quickly and without a second thought the majority of people inevitably jump and say, "To have a child." My next question is: "Why?" I'm really not surprised that most people don't seem to have any specific reason, as our instinct to be loved and have children is wonderful and innately human and not something we need to spend time and effort thinking about.

If I then suggest that we imagine the baby is a done deal and ask, "But what would you love for yourself?", people are also often lost for an answer as their focus has for so many years been almost entirely on becoming a parent. With a little further prompting and encouragement to step outside of the baby "box" people's deeper needs and desires emerge and can be quite surprising. There is often a great sense of relief and excitement in them when they allow themselves to think about something other than conception and the longed-for baby – especially when they realise that this new focus on self could possibly help with their "main complaint".

How often do we stop to ask ourselves what we would truly love in our lives, and question the things we think we want and intend to get? We just get on with life, and our innate talents and desires get mixed in with a whole list of stuff we think we need, or they are forgotten altogether. Regarding the patients I typically see for fertility, it is easy to make the assumption that their primary intention is to have a child almost to the exclusion of everything else in their lives. But if I talk to a couple separately and ask them how they will feel if they are unsuccessful in becoming parents, they will frequently give different responses; one truly devastated, the other taking it in their stride and sure that they will find something else and be fine to go on with life. But is this always the truth?

As we get older and leave the spontaneity of our youth, our "heart's desire" and what we think we "want" both individually and as a couple can become confused, resulting in many mixed messages. This becomes apparent when couples negotiate the difficult path of fertility treatment and try to manage their relationship along the way.

I often see this with men. They say they want a child, but seem indifferent, and appear to be shrugging their shoulders as if they're just along for the ride. I don't think there's much room in our culture for men to be over-enthusiastic about becoming a parent. For women it's an issue that, like it or not, is brought up throughout their lives, from gifts of dolls to pointed remarks about biological clocks and the constant monthly reminder that their system is preparing for a child. Men, who are often ignored in fertility clinics and even registered in their partner's name when giving a semen sample, get more involved as they go along when they have had the time to think about the process and invest in the idea. Often when the first round of IVF fails, for example, men are surprised at how disappointed they feel.

So what is the significance of this magic word "intention" and how does it help when hoping to conceive? And, given what I said earlier about the importance of "not trying" to have a baby, isn't it contradictory to suddenly talk about "intention"?

Teenagers, you might say, get pregnant without intention all the time, but that's not entirely true. For them "intention" is a clear, primitive drive to get out there and seduce and be seduced and make babies. They don't accidentally fall into bed together. It's very spontaneous, very pure and very powerful, and it works also in older couples in the honeymoon period. "Instinct" is perhaps another term for it; the intention that's the driving force in nature to make things happen. It could be argued that "intention" fuels our libido and powers the drive to conceive.

In the Five-Element system the mind or our intelligence is the sum total of all the activities of the organs and functions. When we are in balance our heart and mind are one, and our heart's desire to have a child is programmed and ever present in all of us. This primal code is set to provide the potential for the survival of our species, but the only way this message can be realised is through intention in the holistic sense.

If you are ready to become a parent in your head and on a deeper level your heart is not on board and therefore not in sync, this lack of congruence will jar and could negatively affect the desired outcome. In Chinese philosophy the heart and the uterus are seen as having a very close relationship; the "heart-uterus axis" refers to the heart stimulating ovulation while providing a home and dwelling place for the spirit. Similarly, the uterus becomes the home for the developing child. The ancient Chinese knew that the mind and body alone were not capable of making a baby.

It's taken for granted that generally people want to have children; but, particularly as you get older, the choices you make as you move on from trying naturally, to assisted conception and on again, perhaps, to adoption will involve a change from inexpressed desire to intention. Are you willing to accept this change, acknowledge that where you started is not where you are now? There may come a point in the process when your heart is no longer in it, and you want to turn your focus and the focus of your relationship elsewhere. Does it have to be a child that is biologically both yours and your partner's, or even biologically yours at all?

It's not just about having a strategy, but really engaging with your deeper feelings on the matter. Sometimes the block to conception begins in a misplaced, misjudged intention that you don't really experience consciously at all.

One couple I see, Steve and Cathy, are a good illustration. Steve already has four kids from a previous marriage, who are going through their teens and acting out with a vengeance. He's a very full-on character, with plenty of energy, always at the centre of his social circle. He's hugely happy with Cathy, who's also extremely sociable and cherished by her friends. Neither is fundamentally troubled in themselves or in their relationship; for all Steve's fireworks, they seem to be very content, except for the fact that they have now started on the conveyor belt of fertility treatment.

Steve thinks Cathy wants a child, Cathy says she does too, but I'm not sure that they are prepared to go through what's required. The main physical problem is that both are extremely overweight and don't do any exercise. This is not in itself a guarantee of infertility, but certainly a factor to be considered if there is a problem with conceiving naturally. My first suggestion would be that they change their diets and lifestyles, but they seem to just want to sweep that under the carpet. They want to have acupuncture and then IVF and maybe ICSI, or an egg donor if that doesn't work.

They are disregarding their ambivalence about having a child – highlighted to me by the way they overlook the most glaring obstacle – because they are dazzled by the list of options available to them at various clinics. Why create a problem where none exists? They could go on happily with their lives without changing their weight or their lifestyle, surrounded by friends and family. They could also commit themselves to becoming healthier, and I'm sure they'd conceive then, but at the moment they don't have to take responsibility for their bodies as IVF offers them a distraction and a way to evade their own lack of conviction about having a child at all. For me as a practitioner, success wouldn't necessarily be Cathy getting pregnant; it would be both of them improving their health and getting their bodies in as fine a fettle as their minds and spirits.

In contrast to Cathy and Steve, my patient Eve had a focused intention and willingness to do whatever it takes:

I have a daughter who is now 21, and when she was four I had a second child, a little boy, who sadly died four days after he was born, and we were devastated. He'd had the equivalent of a massive stroke in utero a few days before he was born, but nobody knew why, and we were told to wait eighteen months before trying again.

We were very fortunate to get pregnant again and I had very good care, and my second son was born without problems. Everything was fine, but I still felt as though there was a gap. I didn't need to replace my first son; I just felt very strongly that there was a space for someone else. I didn't act on it, but got on with my career and kept myself busy, but when I was 40 the feeling came back more strongly than ever.

My partner and I talked long and hard about having a fourth child, but when we tried, nothing happened. After a few years I started having acupuncture and within three months I was pregnant, but I had loads of stress at the time – my father and my best friend were dying, and I was racing between them – and I miscarried at two months.

By this time I was 44 or 45 and very aware that I was really pushing it, and running out of time. We decided that the best thing was to give up and to adopt a child, and began the interviews and home tests required. The agency were delighted to have us as mature parents and said that everything should go well when we turned in a huge stack of references. We and the children were interviewed repeatedly and it all went swimmingly until we were within months of being given a child.

The agency called me at work and said there was a problem. In one of the interviews my son had said that he didn't mind what a new child in the family looked like, as long as they didn't act like the very disturbed son of a friend of ours, who was hyperactive. That raised a flag. Just like that, the agency rescinded everything, and we were back where we'd started.

Acupuncture helped keep me sane during all this heartbreak, but I didn't think we had any chance of filling that gap in the family. That was when Gerad suggested using an egg donor. I was still fit and healthy and didn't think I would have a problem carrying a child. I just thought that my eggs were too old, and it would be irresponsible to use them.

Once we'd found a good clinic, everything flew by. In only a few months we were sent details of all the potential donors, which was really quite odd. The clinic was in America and all the women had such glamorous headshots, and it was bizarre, like supermarket shopping. There were lists of their college degrees and so on. You never get a chance to talk to them, and you think you should take a long time choosing, but at the same time you have the clinic telling you that you have to make up your mind by Wednesday!

Eventually we chose a donor and my husband flew to the States to give his sample; he flew in one day, did the business and flew out the next. He said it was the most bizarre thing he'd done in his whole life. Gerad had been treating me to make sure I was in peak condition, and I flew over to have the embryo implanted a few days later, before returning home. I had a very smooth pregnancy and the NHS was brilliant about it. There was no judgment at all, and they were all incredibly supportive. Our son was born nine months later, when I was 50 – this precious, chatty little boy who brings so much joy to all of us.

I never felt weird about adopting or using an egg donor. I love babies, and I love children, and I just didn't feel it would be an issue. I think you have to be a pretty tough person to go through it though, because you're putting yourself through a lot. I already had two healthy children so I could be a teeny bit pragmatic about it, although of course you put all your hopes in. If it's your last option and you have no child, then it must be agony. I would like more people to think they could do this and think it's not only for really wealthy people. I'm lucky I've been able to explore and fulfil that drive I had.

Intention is all about "showing up" for something that is real; being fully present to whatever it is you hope to achieve without the need or desire to "make" it happen. Ambivalence is the opposite. This is a very subtle distinction – ambivalence can get confused with the passive hands-off approach of "Let's just step back and see if it happens", just as showing up for something can get confused with the determined sheer grit approach of "I will succeed". There's no guarantee, for example, of finding a partner just because you think you want one; you have to feel something as you get out in the world and meet people. This is also true of fertility – there are no guarantees of success, but there is a lot you can do, and a clear and congruent relationship between your heart and mind can make an enormous difference to your hopes and dreams of success.

Gratitude

What I see as one of the great obstacles to a peaceful and graceful path to having a child is our Western mindset and culture of "entitlement". We somehow came up with the idea that we are entitled to so many aspects of our life – including a loving partner and children – and when we don't get them as expected we feel abandoned and lost like small children who cry "It's not fair!". This may sound harsh but most of us have been brainwashed by our collectively created consumer culture, which would have us believe that having and owning more and more is a human right, and this only serves to feed our sense of entitlement.

When someone is hoping to conceive, my advice to them is to relax, sit back and remember that we are not entitled to anything. Life and all it brings is a wonderful gift and every day that we wake up and realise we still even exist is a blissful bonus. In our culture of "I want" and "I need", we have lost a genuine sense of gratitude for some of the most basic things in life – health being one.

We take our body and mind for granted when things are working well, and we rarely stop to marvel at this complex organism that is our physical form performing most tasks quietly and efficiently and leaving us alone to get on with life. However, as soon as something goes wrong it becomes overwhelming, gratitude flies out the window and all those years of great health are forgotten. We become spiritually lazy and with this comes unhappiness, sucking us straight down the victim chute.

Not only do we expect a perfect mate but we also want the character we have been sold since childhood, and then when it comes to relationship plus baby, it seems that we get even more particular and generally favour the "Mills and Boon" version as being the best way to have a child. Even some of the most liberal and alternative people I know tone down and suddenly morph into Mr and Mrs 1950s Suburbia when the baby, making alarm bell rings.

By moving out of entitlement and into a place of gratitude for what we have right now (you are still breathing, I hope), we immediately soften and sync with the rhythms of nature that are waiting in the wings to provide the very best for us: nature's gift of abundance.

The Fertility "Business"

Since the first IVF baby was born in 1978, our attitude to conception has become increasingly commercial. Conception used to be a gift – sought or unsought – from nature, and we had to accept what it chose to deal us. Now we can buy a pregnancy, or at least a chance of one, with medical procedures that give us the illusion of control at every stage. In 2010, two vets in Australia even proclaimed that soon no human would need to have sex to procreate; IVF would take care of all that. Cows had a 100 per cent greater chance of conceiving with artificial methods than naturally, they pointed out, and surely the same potential was just a hop, skip and a jump in science away for us humans.

The problem, they admitted, was that for humans, IVF works only in 32.2 per cent of cycles of treatment for women under the age of 35, and as they get older, the success rate drops even lower. The Human Fertilisation and Embryology Association's tally for the overall success rate of all medical fertility clinics is just 22 per cent: less than a quarter. Why doesn't it work as well for humans as it does for cattle? Could it be that we're far more complicated beings than cows? Of course. A cow doesn't worry about its relationship, or ending up on its own in old age, or even if there will be food tomorrow or if it wants to change its job and follow its dreams.

Not surprisingly, these vets overlook what makes us human – as do many of the doctors and gurus in the fertility industry – assuming that a human is so simple that you just have to provide the right fodder and work out the correct schedule, and conception will ensue. Failing that, you can add large amounts of hormones to super-enhance the production of eggs, and then give the sperm a special boost by injecting it directly into the target. No obstacles, no struggle, no natural selection and, of course, no orgasms.

Some consultants seem to think that if modern medicine can't help a couple, it's their own fault, and not that of the fertility business. They will drop bombshells on their patients, telling them they have a low chance, or not a chance in hell, and a lot of these people are plunged into despair, for which there's little or no counselling. I'm not opposed to all the incredible advances that have been made in medical technology, and I am happy to help people who have entered into the process, including those who do have physical or mechanical problems, such as blocked fallopian tubes or extensive endometriosis that cannot be overcome by clearing up their lifestyle or sorting out their hearts. But I still feel that there's a hole at the core of the business. The state of a patient's spirit is too invisible, and if it is visible, it is generally considered too time-consuming and complicated and nuanced for a fertility clinic to tackle.

Sometimes, for the prospective parents, it comes down to a catch 22: leave work on time and take an hour or two to relax and recover and balance work and life on the chance that it will help you conceive, or else work those longer hours so you can afford the conveyor belt of treatment and a trip overseas to find an egg donor, all the time with this drumbeat telling you "too late, hurry, hurry!"

Added to the purely physical interpretation of fertility problems is a culture of blame that thrives on scare stories and the cult of the biological clock. These warnings to women to conceive before it's "too late" are usually accompanied by some science-y statistics that don't hold up well on closer examination. One headline screams that most women have lost seven-eighths of their 2,000,000 eggs by the age of 30. If you do the maths, you realise that this average woman still has 500,000 eggs to spare at 30 – even octomom doesn't need to have 500,000 babies. You need only one egg to have a child, not an omelette's worth.

Part of the problem is the widespread belief that at birth, a baby girl contains a full set of eggs, ready to start rolling down the fallopian tubes at puberty, and that, if they're not used early enough, then just like chicken eggs in a fridge they will "go off". This is nonsense. You are born with the potential for a certain number of eggs. The quality of those eggs depends on the quality of your overall health at the time that the egg receives the hormonal signal to mature, prior to erupting from the ovary and heading down the fallopian tubes to your womb.

Some women are told they have too many "natural killer cells" in their uterus, which might be attacking implanted foetuses. Enterprising doctors then suggest a dose of drugs that will knock out their immune system for a while, so the killer cells can't gobble up the new embryo. There is no conclusive proof that uterine natural killer cells do attack embryos, or even that the blood test performed for this "diagnosis" provides an accurate reflection of the number of marauding cells in the womb, but of course it sounds dramatic, and I'm sure it terrifies women who are told they are harbouring baby-killing organisms!

A few years ago clinics began to trumpet a new test, for anti-Müllerian hormone levels (AMH), which they said would "predict a woman's menopause" by telling her how many eggs she had left. The result of this, for me, was a flurry of devastated women in my clinic who'd been told they had far too few ova left to conceive.

One woman who, at 41, hadn't conceived after two years (a pretty normal span of time, all things considered) went to a one-stop-shop clinic, which told her that they would just run some tests. She had no idea what most of them were, and when her results came in, the consultant "gleefully" announced that her AMH level was so low that there was no way she would conceive naturally, so they'd put her straight on the clinic's egg-sharing programme. When she expressed her horror and shock, the doctor snapped back, "Well, what do expect when you're over 40?"

She was furious and left immediately, later booking an appointment to begin a course of acupuncture. After six months she had conceived naturally, without any help from the consultant. She believes now that it was a direct result of the acupuncture treatment at our clinic, but I think this may have played only a small role because, aside from her understandable anger with the consultant, she had a healthy, balanced life and outlook. If it took you, say, six months to conceive in your early twenties, that's six rolls of the dice; three years to conceive at 41 is 36 rolls – it may only have been a matter of holding her nerve until the right number came up and the right egg met the right sperm.

Faith had her first child at 36 with no difficulty, but when she got pregnant with her second child three years later, she miscarried at eleven weeks, which shocked her. She lost some of her confidence in her ability to have a child, and when her husband lost his job and slid into depression, she became increasingly anxious that she would never have another child.

As she'd been told that her greatest chance of conceiving was in the first few months immediately after miscarriage, and as her husband was not mentally in the right place to enthusiastically start making babies, she decided to have an AMH test in order to understand "how long she had left".

The verdict was a 0.3 per cent chance. Faith was gutted. She went from being a capable, outwardly successful woman to a wreck, and by the time she came to the clinic she had lost half her hair and was running hysterically back and forth between nutritionists, reflexologists and me. The only time I've seen such a dramatic depression resulting from a medical diagnosis is in the newly diagnosed HIV patients of the early 1990s whom I treated at Kings College Hospital. It felt like a death sentence to her. She still had her husband, her home and her daughter, and there was no proof other than the AMH test to say that she couldn't have another child, but it was as though she could barely hear what was being said to her.

I have never seen a contraceptive placebo as powerful as a low AMH result, delivered without sympathy. Faith went from a woman who had conceived easily twice in her late thirties – supposedly with this 0.3 per cent chance – to "barren". Hopefully, it will be possible for her to regain the equilibrium and health she had before she took the test.

The AMH test doesn't tell you the quality of the eggs that remain, only the quantity. It's also inconsistent – if a woman has more than one AMH test she may get a completely different result each time. Plenty of women who've been told their eggs are inadequate have gone on to have absolutely no problems conceiving, while others who've had a positive tick on their clipboard have found themselves having difficulty.

As for sperm testing, this can be equally fraught with inconsistencies. A sample is taken and the sperm examined under the microscope. How many are there? Are they swimming well? Are they damaged? An assessment is made and the verdict delivered. The man is either given the thumbs-up, or emasculated by being told he's the one at fault.

The problem is that it takes sperm three months to mature from first development to ejaculation. In the testicles the naive sperm cells are constantly creating new gametes. Ideally, these will go on growing and developing their tails and nice healthy heads until a batch of 40,000,000 is ready to go a quarter of a year later. In reality, the entire process, even before the sperm are anywhere near a vagina, is natural selection. The cells are very sensitive to their environment, so if, say, you celebrated the New Year to the full on December

31st, the sperm that began their lives that day might have been dealt a severe early blow, and struggle. In any case, only 10 per cent of the 40,000,000 have a head that's strong enough to break the walls of the ovum, and only 10 per cent of those have a tail. That leaves 400,000 and some of those don't have any genetic material in the head. And then they face that hostile environment, with an inimical pH level and all those phagocyte cells. Oh, and if the man took his test at the end of March, those soused New Year sperm will give an unfairly poor rating. Perhaps he did a two-week detox at the beginning of January. If the clinic tested his sperm again in early April, they might find the microscope slide full of sturdy specimens, and give the same man a clean bill of fertility health.

Worse still, a man with a spectacularly unhealthy lifestyle might happen to have his test three months after a rare dose of sobriety and restraint, with the end result that he unfairly gets the all-clear and his female partner has to go through years of hormonal injections and examinations to work out what's wrong with her. This is Martin's story:

One of the first things that was suggested when I went for acupuncture treatment was that I should be tested for a change, and to have three tests over a period of two months. When we got all the results back it turned out that the problem had been with me all along. I wish that could have been identified earlier because we would have saved ourselves a lot of heartache and waiting. All of the waiting and not knowing takes an emotional toll and it takes a toll on your relationship too. If I could give any advice to men in the same situation I found myself in, it would be to try to prevent the medical focus being just on the woman. I'm sure men feel the same as women who have been told they are infertile – that it's some sort of failure of their sexuality if they can't produce a child – and in some ways the medical profession lets them off the hook by concentrating on women. So the men don't have to confront what's going on, and can avoid awkward soul-searching. It's not like men are going to be rushing into internet forums to talk about their low sperm counts! It may feel like there's a lot stacked against taking a holistic perspective, but you have to consider that something is up with you, and take steps to do something, because a lot of implications can follow from the way you're treated. We might have had more children if we'd had that clarity earlier on.

Too often, in my view, women are bombarded with this message that it's all their fault. They're selfish if they have babies as teenagers, and selfish if they wait till their forties, selfish if they only have one child, selfish if they have more than three, selfish if they have a high-flying career, selfish if they don't earn enough to support the children. They're using up NHS resources if they have IVF, and state resources if they have a large family. They're told to settle for "Mr Good Enough" instead of holding out for a consuming passion. Ageism and misogyny are packaged in emotive terms like "Russian roulette".

Once you have children, as Lizzie put it, "Everything you do is wrong. I stayed at home with my son because I could work from there and he was so precious to me, but as soon as people find out I only have one child they disapprove. When I was growing up, if your mother went out to work it was the same thing. If you have children too young, too late, too quickly, not quickly enough – people pass comment. It's all rubbish and you have to steer your own course. Every family is different."

Similarly, a childless life is often cast as a sad, wasted one. For those like me who have no kids, that comes as a bit of a surprise, and it's also pretty insulting to be told that your life counts for nothing compared to that of those who have managed to produce a child. Your relation-ships, your loves, your home, your career, your contribution to the world, the sum of you as an individual is truly nothing if you haven't had a child? It's a doubtful kind of world to want to live in.

As we've seen in this book, by the time a lot of people

reach their later thirties, they no longer understand what "normal" and "healthy" might be for them as they're entrenched in habits or a lifestyle that their body can no longer sustain while simultaneously nourishing a pregnancy. Once that imbalance is corrected, be it physical, mental or spiritual, many "older" women and men go on to conceive. From what I've seen, as long as a woman is menstruating and a man producing sperm, they have a chance to conceive. Why else would nature expend the resources on a menstrual cycle and sperm production? If it can happen naturally, then why judge? If there is a "time bomb" it's the risk we take with our spiritual and physical health overall – not just our genitals and reproductive organs – by not being able to stand back and set ourselves straight.

Success

One of the greatest difficulties in treating patients for infertility is that there is only one perceived successful outcome – a baby. No matter how much I communicate the other benefits of treatment, patients tend to come for one specific reason and this is where their focus remains. This is, of course, completely understandable but the job of the acupuncturist is to support and care for all patients equally and there will always be the patients who are not successful in having a child and should not be seen as having failed. The stakes are high for all patients struggling with infertility. It is a very public experience and people feel compelled to succeed for not only their own needs and desires but also the needs and desires of family and friends who have their own set of expectations.

Dorothy's story is indicative of the subjective nature of success:

I've been trying for almost two years to have a second child. I was diagnosed in my early thirties with polycystic ovary syndrome, and my GP told me it would take three years to conceive a child so we started trying as soon as we were married. Within three months I fell pregnant – aged 34 – and we were totally gobsmacked and delighted. I had a very healthy pregnancy, but our daughter's birth was very difficult, and I caught a very rare strep C septicaemia infection – I think I was the only woman in the country to have it – and nearly died. My organs were on the verge of failure and layers of skin came off my hands and feet like a snake. I had to have blood transfusions and the doctors threatened a hysterectomy, although I didn't have to have one in the end. When I got out of the hospital six and a half weeks later, the doctors told me to leave it at least a year before trying to conceive a second child, to give my body a chance to recover.

When we first started trying again, I was very stressed for the first six months. Part of it was that I desperately wanted to have a normal birth, and I never wanted my daughter to think that it was because I nearly died having her that she didn't have a brother or sister. A lot of people said they couldn't believe I was even considering going through it all again, but for me it felt as though I would mend something by having a second child.

After nine months, nothing seemed to be happening and I panicked that the infection had done some permanent damage. I went to my GP but she brushed me off and said, "You'll be absolutely fine." Luckily, as I had private insurance I was able to begin a series of tests, but I also started seeing Gerad for acupuncture at the same time, to see if that would help.

For the first four months, I was still stressed out. The medical results were coming in and revealing that there was nothing wrong with my husband or me, and to be honest that just made it all the more frustrating. Every time I got my period, I'd have a bad few days when the horm-ones were in full flow and I just didn't get it – what was wrong? Why weren't we getting pregnant? And then you just think, onwards and upwards, into the next month!

Acupuncture helped with that. I also started to see a therapist at the same time, and gradually I've got a much more balanced perspective. Now I just want to follow this journey with a more laissez-faire attitude and just let things happen. After each session there is definitely a change in me. I feel very upbeat when I come out of the clinic; it feels like a total release.

We haven't conceived naturally as a result of the treatment, but I do feel like I'm a better person for it, and my husband would definitely say I'm less stressed. I would never have done all this work on myself if we'd been able to have a second child without a hitch, and I think I'm going to be a better mother to my daughter because I'm stronger now and I'm dealing with my issues.

I do still want a sibling for my girl because I had three sisters and we're all incredibly close, and it's hard to think of her missing out on having that kind of support and friendship. We're embarking on IVF now, and on our first trip to the clinic I felt so much less alone. Suddenly we were surrounded by people who were going through the same thing.

I don't regret not trying IVF sooner, because I'm in a much better frame of mind than I was a year ago before I started seeing the therapist and having acupuncture. I think it would have been horrendous, and hell on the whole family as well, and I wouldn't have been prepared for the fact that it might just not work. It's a formidable prospect because I don't know how the drugs will affect me or if we shouldn't try one more time to have a child naturally, but I feel proud that we lasted two years and didn't just leap in after a few months. It just feels like the right point on our journey, and we'll deal with it as it comes.

In the West we have a relatively fixed idea of good or bad, success or fail, which feels unyielding and restrictive at times. When I first started treating patients for infertility, I was also sucked into this success/fail paradigm, which was exciting when treatment resulted in a pregnancy and dispiriting when it didn't. I quickly realised that this pressure and my own emotional investment in success did not serve my patients. My expectations only created more pressure for them.

Life is gentler than this, and, providing we have a good level of mental and spiritual flexibility, what we see as success or failure can just simply be our current state, which is neither "good" nor "bad" but just a fact. True balance and harmony have no "rub", do not seek to compartmentalise and label people, situations or aspirations.

There are, of course, those clients who leave disappointed, upset, even angry – they had high hopes.

Grief follows – a clear sense of the child who was going to arrive in your life and now never will. Jennifer said, "I was absolutely furious when we stopped trying, but as time went on ultimately I realised I have done everything I could. I've accepted it now."

For any of you who have not experienced this kind of loss, it is hard to describe the depth of pain and devastation that some people feel. It is a strange and isolating bereavement, as nothing tangible has been lost other than a thought, a hope, a dream and possibly an expectation. One of the great coping strategies for most people is to move out of grief and victimhood by recognising this truth – it was just a thought. Jennifer also coped: "If you're not given the gift of a child it doesn't mean you're not deserving, or that someone else who was given one is more deserving than you. It's just the way life is. There's no big force maliciously excluding you."

This is Andrea's story.

My husband and I wanted to start having children when we got engaged, but decided to hold off until we were married. Quite soon after our wedding, I was diagnosed with an autoimmune disorder called Graves' disease and had to take a course of medication that ruled out trying for a baby in the meantime, as it would have been dangerous for both me and the foetus. I'd been going back and forth to my GP with symptoms for a long time, and it was frustrating how long it took to diagnose the very classic symptoms I had. He kept saying I must have a virus, or early-onset rheumatism. After I finished these drugs I had radiation therapy, which of course meant I had to delay trying for a baby once more.

Eventually I was moved to a prescription drug that allowed me to conceive and be pregnant without the baby or I coming to harm, but nothing happened, so of course we found ourselves in the long, tedious process of doing the rounds of more doctors and more tests. Finally they said, "We don't know what's wrong, but you'll probably need IVF and there's a year's waiting list." Mercifully, we were able to go privately, and start the IVF process earlier.

I hated IVF. The first cycle felt like a last resort. It was where you went when you couldn't conceive naturally. That was just how I saw it and I was very nervous about the whole process; it was daunting. I'd sit in the waiting room and look at all the other women and think, "I don't want to be here, I don't want to be another woman in an IVF clinic."

I had no sense of sisterhood or solidarity. I thought this was just something I'd go through and then I'd have a child and it would all be behind me, but this rage and anger was amplified by the fact that all my friends were getting pregnant, taking maternity leave and pushing babies around in prams. As each person, one by one, announced their pregnancy, I could just see that statistically I was going to be the one who didn't have a kid.

It was a really dark time for me, and I did start seeing a psychotherapist, although I'm not sure quite what I got out of it other than that it took the pressure off my husband and saved my marriage. My husband was unhappy because I was depressed, and I was just leaning on him, and the best thing about the shrink was that it got me to take all that sadness out of the house and have somebody else to talk to so he didn't have to prop me up all the time. I probably got more self-knowledge and tools but I stopped going after a few years because I saw that I could be going to see her for ever and ever! She was trying to get me to accept the fact that I might never have biological children, but that was just inconceivable to me. It was inconceivable that they should be inconceivable!

I started having acupuncture appointments with Gerad at this time and went five or six times, but in the end I gave up because I was just overwhelmed by everything I was going through, and the acupuncture just felt like another thing that was reminding me that I wasn't getting pregnant. I couldn't see it as part of the solution. I was already pissed off that I had to have even more treatment after all I'd been through with Graves' disease. It just seemed like more needles being stuck into me; part of the problem, rather than a solution. I was very angry with the world about everything.

We went through six cycles of IVF in four years, five with fresh embryos and one with a frozen one. I started having treatment with Gerad again later, and it helped to calm me down and reduce the old stomach-churning anxiety. It's a cliché but after a session I'd feel like something had lifted. I don't know if it was the needles or the calm atmosphere at the clinic or the fact that I took it far more seriously than the therapy sessions, but it alleviated the very physical anxiety I felt.

Despite that, none of the implantations have worked out. I thought that IVF was one of those things you did and you were pregnant in no time, because I didn't know anyone who'd gone through it. Now I understand what a gamble it is, personally and financially each time you do it, and we're just about ready to give up. I know it's hard for my husband because he couldn't really do anything, and he would just have to watch this big bag of drugs arrive for me and then me subjecting myself to the whole procedure and it's horrible when it doesn't work. Now we're looking seriously at adopting, and I haven't had any further goes at IVF for eight months.

It's really hard to give up, though. I'm 39, and I wonder, if it worked this time, I'd have a baby in just nine months. It's not even about having our own biological children; it's just about the amount of days till we can hold our child and have a family. When you've already been waiting for years, through all these delays, it's incredibly hard to give up. Adoption will take at least two years, and it feels like once more we're back at the drawing board, at the beginning of yet another process with new things to fathom and understand, but my friends who have adopted are right: at least you know there's a child at the end of it, unlike IVF.

The last time we went to a fertility clinic to hear the results of tests to work out why the IVF had failed, we were almost excited because we thought finally a doctor would tell us that they'd found the problem and we definitely couldn't have biological children, and then we would go on and adopt without a backward glance. In the end they said what they always said: that we were healthy, my eggs had a full set of chromosomes, and that we should try again. It actually felt like bad news.

When we've marked a year without medical fertility treatment, we can begin the process of adoption. The acupuncture and chat I've had with Gerad since that last trip to the IVF clinic has been all about balancing me and thinking about what life will be like without my own birth children, and just concentrating on making me a happier and less stressed person above all. I'm going to need to make some changes to my life, like perhaps finding a new career, because though I love my job it stresses me out. The important thing is to know that we have lots of options and that everything is open. I've now realised that not having a kid is not the only reason why I'm unhappy and anxious so much of the time. I can't rely on getting pregnant to make myself a happy person. I have to take responsibility for being happier. There's more to life than having biological children, and you can't control everything in your world. It's taken a long time for me to get to a place where I can accept that I won't carry and give birth to my own children; it was just too painful to imagine for a long time, and it was something that I'd assumed always, always, always, would happen for us. We don't want to go into adoption thinking it's the second-best thing, just with some trepidation. I do feel quite confident and positive about it in a way that I didn't feel a year ago. I don't think, "Oh poor me, what more do I have to go through?" I think, "Blimey, this is going to be hectic but really exciting." It's finally something positive, and when I hear stories about people who have adopted kids, I just think it's amazing and so lovely.

Now there's a part of me that can go down that hippy route and think maybe we weren't supposed to have our own children because there are some children out there who need us like we need them. Matt and I need a family, and those children need a family, and we just need to come together.

This was Jack's experience:

I went in for acupuncture initially to try and change my infertility. Then at a certain point I thought, "Acupuncture isn't working for my fertility, but it's certainly working for the rest of my life." I wasn't upset that I didn't have a cure, but I was glad I got something out of it for my general well-being. One positive outcome of my infertility was that it forced my wife and I to tackle issues in our relationship that we hadn't quite dealt with up till then. It made us sit down and re-evaluate what we wanted and how we worked together. We needed to be really close and really aligned and connected to proceed in having kids in a way that was going to be much more difficult and challenging than we'd expected.

There's this whole guy thing about passing on your name. Fortunately, it was never that important to me, but I understand if you feel like something's dying out with you; to be honest, though, once you have your kids and they're walking around and talking and doing things with you, I don't think it matters very much.

Our eldest child is a donor insemination baby, and my wife carried him and gave birth to him. After he was born she got pregnant in the same way with sperm from the same donor, but miscarried, after which we learnt that she would be unable to have any more children. It was an incredibly difficult time, to take a second major diagnosis like this, but I think the fact that we'd been through it before with me helped. It seemed easier to move on to adoption for our second child.

It took two years at least, and just when we'd given up on it ever happening, we were told there was a three-month-old baby for us to adopt. Adoption is difficult and it's hit and miss with a lot of uncertainty because they're not sure if they'll have a kid for you and then, suddenly, boom! Three weeks later you take him home. It's crazy. It's crazy emotionally and practically but that's what it is, and it's amazing.

We tried everything, and we've experienced it all, but we also got the family that was in our vision. It took a lot of grief and pain and sadness, but it doesn't really matter how you get them once they're running around your house.

People think if they have a birth child they'll know what they'll get, but they won't! There are a lot of issues – physical or mental – that a kid can have, whether you adopt them or conceive them naturally. Having kids is a crapshoot, and will ever be thus. Children are not really yours anyway. They're their own people and they're going to run off eventually – you just have them for a while. It's what all biological parents end up having to learn, but when you have an adopted child, you know it from the start and can give them space to be themselves.

Sometimes our options are restricted by a set of circumstances beyond our control, such as, for example, an intractable physical problem that makes conception impossible, as it was for Jack. When this happens, we have to make allowances and work within those restrictions, but we should always avoid making false restrictions for ourselves. Life requires us to be flexible, and sometimes we have to change our goals and what we're reaching for too.

Kate was a big hitter in a government department when she met her partner, Bruno, in her late twenties, and they'd been happily together for several years before she arrived at the clinic looking for help with having a baby. She was very dynamic, and very ambitious at work, and one of the things she told me in the first consultation was that she had never considered having children, but now she'd been made to realise that she had to think about it now, or else miss an opportunity. There was a sudden wave of pressure from family and friends wanting to know when they'd have children, with the general consensus being that no job and no marriage could be so enthralling that it would be as satisfying as having kids. They were both from big families. She'd been told that once she had a baby in her arms she'd feel differently. She'd spoken with Bruno and they'd decided to go for it, but you couldn't mistake their ambivalence. They had developed a certain determination, however although it felt like a box-ticking exercise, a challenge that they had taken on for the sake of it. She rallied and got fully behind it, but it wasn't happening.

I thought she was great. She was one of those genuinely strong people who are well in their own skin; she was not suffering from any kind of spiritual crisis. There was nothing really wrong with her and she wasn't in denial about anything, except perhaps this ambivalent attitude to conceiving. Kate wasn't interested in the idea that maybe it wouldn't happen if she didn't want it deep down, and now that it was becoming a challenge, she wanted to overcome it as she'd overcome problems at work. "I'll just get on with it and see what happens," she told me.

After two years, the baby project was heading towards "failure". Bruno had become so caught up in the process that he was making charts and timing their sex life, and their previously close-knit relationship was suffering under the strain. The whole thing had started to be very uncomfortable, and I felt as though I was treating her just in an effort to stop her falling into this self-created problem. They'd set themselves up for failure in something they had never really cared about much in the first place. I questioned my own ability to treat her because I was treating something that wasn't there. I just wanted to keep her as strong as she was when she arrived for the first consultation.

Suddenly she disappeared for a few months and I wondered what had happened. Then she was back at the clinic again, telling me that she had quit her job. She and Bruno were going to move back to his home country of Italy and set up a nursery for local children. They'd started using contraception again and didn't want to have children.

Why on earth did she want to work with kids then?

I asked, and she said she just wanted a business and she loved being around kids, even if she was happy to go home without them at the end of the day. What had first seemed bizarre was actually a perfect ending: it was clean, satisfactory and sorted. It was a huge life change, but they've been there for five years now and are thriving. I sometimes wonder what would have happened if she had conceived, but in the end just the idea of a baby was enough to create the opportunity for an incredible life change and fresh challenges.

The Gift

We live in a world of good and bad, light and shade, war and peace; a world of duality where nothing is static and which exists only by virtue of this ever-present tension. What we witness in nature is a sophisticated complex system in constant flow, moving between chaos and order but always returning to a state of balance.

The human spirit is part of the same force that makes all life possible and which directs nature and the natural world around us, bringing us back to our true selves. I've tried to explain how, in Taoist philosophy, we are part of nature, born of it, maintained by it and subject to its laws, and that trusting our spirit's guidance and strength is fundamental to us. We need to be in a relationship with spirit and work from this place, so that rather than strive in the world to find peace, we start from peace as we strive.

We all have the capacity to be healthy, content and productive human beings. Even after years of depression or health problems we still have that positive potential. A seed can lie dormant for years waiting for the conditions to be right and then have the energy to sprout.

You can choose from a great array of practitioners and books and services to help you in the process, but none of us can fix you, ultimately. I don't believe that fertility gurus exist. There are people who are prepared to serve and help others and there are people who share wisdom. They are ordinary people who give good advice. They can help you discover a way forward, and a way to negotiate emotional and physical changes, but without your own efforts to listen to yourself, their assistance will go nowhere. Fixing you is your responsibility — although we practitioners and therapists can help when that responsibility feels too much to bear.

Our role is to give you a sense of perspective if you need it, to help you stand back and take a good, subjective look at your life, your thoughts and feelings and to see what drives them. Are you in touch with your true underlying instinct or sense of self, or are you pursuing/battling for something that you don't want deep down? It's a cliché to say "be yourself" and one whose true meaning is barely understood. All I can do as a practitioner is try to help to bring balance and harmony and hopefully witness the truth revealed. An imbalance in the elements – wood, fire, earth, metal or water – is only one of the ways in which the "knot" manifests itself.

I do believe that we all have the ability to change, but change is difficult. By the time we have left our childhood, struggled through puberty and found our way in the world, we have created our own personal reality. Our friendships, sexual relationships, career paths, personal ideologies and morality form the foundation of the personal perspective that frames our life experience. What we perceive through these windows appears to be real and fixed. For some of us the view is pleasant and easy, for others it is difficult and troubled but it is our view and of our making, based on our reactions to the outside world. Faced with a traumatic event in our lives, we have a choice in how we react and what we do with this experience. This event could be used to back up an already crystallised view that life is painful and difficult. Conversely, the experience could be seen as an opportunity to learn and change our core beliefs and perspective. I am not making a judgment about what is the right or wrong way; I am merely suggesting that we have choice and that our choices will affect our future.

In the context of fertility, there is the story of the victim who gets to blame something or someone else, and the story of the brave survivor who battles on in the face of childlessness and is just "fine". Both of these stories come from the negative part of us which is invested in pain and suffering, one which converts pain into a kind of pride and face-saving exercise. These stories do nothing to help us reach fulfilment because they trap us – either in a passive role (the specialists will do it all) or by defining us by a single failure. The third story is that of the person who knows their self and the truth, and draws on their own resources to roll with the punches or to appreciate the good times when they come. When you can be yourself you are empowered; there are no obstacles to your natural inclinations, your personality – your spirit.

It really comes down to how much personal responsibility you are prepared to take, although few people understand what that really means. It doesn't mean being a captain of industry with 200 employees under you and the buck stopping at your desk. It means owning your own feelings and thoughts, and being a person who is accountable to your Self. Our best resources are found inside us – we already have everything we need.

This book is full of stories of people who were pleasantly surprised to discover that the life they'd thought they wanted wasn't necessarily the best for them after all. They left desirable jobs, quit their nice houses, even left the country and began doing something completely different, or found children who needed them to be their parents. There are also stories of people who stopped competing and searching and started to enjoy the life they already had. And once they all discovered their own unique truth, they settled and let life unfold with or without children.

When confronted with something as emotive as believing that we might not be able to have our own child, an opportunity arises. We realise that we are not perfect; and what a gift that is. As Leonard Cohen says in his moving song "Anthem", "There is a crack in everything / That's how the light gets in."

Tools for Balance

The "tools" listed below are based on the advice I have given the countless "baby-making" people I have tried to help over the past 20 years. They are tried and tested, and from the feedback I have received they appear to have been enormously beneficial in helping people reach their goal. They are all based on common sense and will not necessarily be new to you, but implementing them on a daily basis possibly will be. I strongly encourage you to give them a try.

1. Drinking Water

Have you ever sat by a large body of water and listened to the sound? Even gentle rolling waves can sound like four jumbo jets flying overhead. Next time you are at the beach, listen. You will hear not only the relentless and powerful sound of waves dragging the sand backwards and forwards, but an echo of greatness that fills the entire space. The immense power of oceans and rivers can be totally overwhelming, as we have seen in recent years with the tsunamis that have devastated human life in a matter of minutes, and so unsurprisingly we see this awe-inspiring force of nature as something outside of ourselves. Not so.

We are primarily made of space, but after that, the majority of our physical form is water – around 75 per cent of our body mass – and this is the same water you see in the sea, the rain, the snow and the sweat on your forehead, recycled and shared among every living thing in the Earth's atmosphere. We are powerful beings! It's astonishing to realise that the water you drank this morning (if you did, of course) is the same water that dinosaurs were quenching their thirst on millions of years ago.

Water is the origin of life as we know it. We are born of water, grow from water and are sustained throughout our lives by water. All of the attributes of water we witness in nature are present in us – droughts creating dry skin and constipation, fast-flowing rivers delivering hormones and flushing in new ideas, tsunamis producing searing headaches and panic attacks, mountain-top lakes bringing freshness – and a peace of mind.

As we get older we lose our ability to retain water – we dry up – and along with this natural dehydrating process that will eventually take us to our graves, we lose the vital and essential energy that created us in the first place, that powers our life and our ability to contribute to the creation of new life. The power of conception and creation which feeds and divides every cell is rooted in this element and it is no coincidence that it is stronger and more abundant when we are young. I can remember in my teens, twenties and early thirties never drinking any water. Why would I? I never felt thirsty and rarely felt tired. Not only that, late nights, alcohol and emotional chaos didn't seem to stop most of us from conceiving and producing beautiful bouncing babies. Oh, but we were young. As much as it might be fashionable and comforting to shy away from the truth that conception is easier in young people, we must face reality. The good news is that from my experience of helping the chronically dehydrated over-thirties with fertility problems, age is not so much of a concern but proper hydration is.

As I have explained, the role of water is not just to moisturise; it is nature's medicine. Water lubricates, brings power, cleanses, promotes movement, strengthens, balances, dilutes, provides buoyancy... the list goes on. It is nothing short of miraculous and yet many of my patients often complain when I tell them what I think might be the cause of all their problems – inadequate consumption of water – they say they are not thirsty. If I bottled it and sold it as an infertility cure I would most likely have enormous success and become a millionaire overnight. People trawl the web looking for the next best substance to ingest in their quest for premium health and optimum fertility and yet their foundation is not in place. For many of us, our body gave up asking for water years ago after we managed to convince it there was a massive drought and to make do with what it had.

I feel so passionately about this that I will go as far as to say that everything – and I mean everything – is dependent on this element. Every new treatment, every new habit, every new strategy you employ to conceive will ultimately fail unless you give yourself this fundamental source of life. From an acupuncture point of view it's essential. The acupuncture needles can move the formless energy in the channels, but this action needs to filter down to the material level, and this is water. Water is the basis of blood, which in turn feeds our muscles, our tendons and ligaments, our skin, our reproductive organs – every part of us.

"My doctor told me I get enough water from food and drinks," one patient protested. "It just won't go down, I can't swallow it," another said, having told me he drinks three pints of beer every night. "It doesn't taste of anything," she complained, "and it's too cold." "But wine and whiskey are made of water!" he said looking at me suspiciously – and so the protests and excuses go on and on. All of the above may be true but what we do know is that dehydration is life threatening and by extension, "new-life threatening". The debate continues and all the fertility experts have their own ideas about water. Become your own expert then – spend some time in nature and see what happens when water is abundant.

2. Eating Breakfast

"Breakfast like a king or queen." Yes – it's as simple as that! We are designed by nature to transform food into life-giving energy between the hours of 7am and 9am. An imaginative and colourful list of excuses, much like the one I described for not drinking water, is conjured up when I encourage people to eat a big breakfast. It would be amusing if the people protesting were not the ones who are hoping to create new life.

I do understand that if it is something you have never done, it will feel strange at first. Your stomach deprived of its primary function for over 30 years is suddenly asked to perform, and of course, it goes into shock. So start simply with bite-size chunks and wean yourself gently in until you are truly feasting every morning. Remember the Law of Midday-Midnight and how ignoring this natural law to eat at this time can disrupt every action for the remainder of your day.

MENU OF THE DAY

- Breakfast like a king or queen – fats, carbohydrates and protein
- Lunch like a prince or princess – carbohydrates and protein
- Dine like a pauper – protein

3. True Rest

We're all very busy – running around, working, socialising, jumping up and down, having sex, travelling, cleaning – you name it, we're doing it. Yet, rest and downtime are often very low on our agenda of important daily activities. Understandably – there's a lot to do.

Doing nothing is often considered a "waste of time" and the idea that we could just sit in a chair and do nothing for an hour is not only verging on sinful but for some of us impossible. The Western work ethic is still strong in many of us despite the decline of its righteous roots, and like all habits, the habit of busy-ness is hard to break when our culture congratulates us for every extra hour we keep ourselves "turned on".

Providing we have a relatively good night's rest, a lie-in on a Sunday and a couple of weeks on a beach somewhere once in a while, we consider we've had enough "down time". The truth is that most of us are deeply tired and running on empty. One of the ways I make a diagnosis when working as an acupuncturist is to read the "pulses" of a patient to establish the strength and the balance of their energy. It amazes me that some people are even able to make it to my treatment room, let alone do all the things I've listed above. The problem we face is that we are not aware of how exhausted we really are. I mentioned earlier in the book the frog in the pot that slowly gets cooked without even knowing the heat's on. The same is true here but the other way round. We get used to our low reserves and compensate with substances, adrenaline and sheer grit. Sometimes we are like a car, whose petrol tank may be near empty but it keeps running at full speed – until it stops. Maintaining an efficient menstrual cycle, maturing eggs and sperm, conceiving and making a baby all take a lot of energy. Make sure "you put a tiger in your tank".

Here are my tips for getting good rest and building your reserves:

- Observe good sleep hygiene. The bedroom is for sex and sleep only. Don't hang out in there, reading, watching TV or chatting on the phone.

- Be asleep by 11pm. You will remember the Chinese Clock that teaches us the importance of getting to bed early and being asleep by 11pm. Start the natural sleep cycles, essential for your regeneration, on time. This will in turn benefit all your organs and the functions that follow for the rest of the 24-hour cycle.

- Get up at the same time every day. Choose a time to get up (ideally no later than 7am) and stick to it every day. There is room for some flexibility but the more routine your body is given, the better quality of sleep you will enjoy.

- Take time to sit – meditate. Sitting or meditating is a great bridge between our unconscious and conscious states. Getting up and immediately rushing around, listening to the radio, checking emails is not the best way to start the day. Sitting or meditating for ten minutes soon after waking is a wonderful way to bring the restful and peaceful state of sleep into the waking day. Sit quietly and focus on the in-breath and the out-breath and put your attention on the stillness that exists within you and away from the busy-ness of your mind. Repeat this throughout the day – even five minutes is enough.

- Be mindful in all you do. This is an extension of the sitting-meditative practice described above. It simply means being fully present and more conscious of your life as it unfolds. It is easy to be distracted by thoughts and spend the whole day in your head. It's exhausting. Take each activity as it comes and try to be fully present to it without judgment. Brushing your teeth is just as valid as securing the next big deal.

- Find an activity that brings you "true rest". "True rest" is not necessarily about going to sleep or napping. We all have something we do that we recognise is good for us. I enjoy taking my dog for a walk, or going for a swim, and I'm aware that after these activities I feel better. It's very subjective and it is important that you decide which ones works for you. Some people find reading books brings "true rest", for others it's stressful. Whatever it is, become aware of it and integrate it into your life as a priority. The quality of all your other activities will immediately improve.

4. The Pendulum

The pendulum is a wonderful transformational tool – simple and extremely effective.

Our thoughts and feelings are in a constant state of flux – impermanent, changeable, sometimes volatile and often unpredictable. They can swing wildly from one polarity to the next, from high to low, joyful to sad, before landing somewhere in between. Imagine your thoughts and feelings as the weight of a pendulum, swinging from side to side. In anyone in a state of good health, when a happy event occurs, or they have a joyful thought, the weight swings towards the "high", and then, once this feeling is acknowledged, it naturally gravitates back to the midpoint – the calm. Maybe a friend of theirs loses a parent, or perhaps they fall and hurt themselves... the pendulum's weight heads to the "low", but once again, when the feelings have been resolved, it heads back to the calm. And so it goes on, constantly moving from one appropriate response to the next.

The reality, however, for most of us is very different; we get stuck or become attached to one side of the pendulum or the other – we have preferences, more often than not favouring the high, but also, at times, favouring the low. The "compulsive swingers", of course, love the ride so much they swing madly from one side to the other, rarely visiting the midpoint or the calm at all.

The purpose of the pendulum as a "tool" is to develop an awareness of how our thoughts and feelings can take over and control our lives. We generally tend to keep the swing to one side or the other because we believe that we are caught in a world that only offers us an either/or option. The pendulum teaches us we can have both.

By climbing up the shaft of the pendulum like a monkey scaling a tree, we realise that there is less and less movement the higher we go. So we can think or feel high or low – and still experience the calm. We spend our lives clinging to the base of the pendulum cooking up strategies to keep us in one place or another but actually none of this stuff seems so important or pressing when you're viewing it from the top. For there, at the pivot, we are in absolute calm, at peace in ourselves and blissfully free of the ephemeral, changing reality going on below.

The golden rule of the pendulum is that you should never make a decision or take action unless you are at the midpoint. By all means enjoy the experience of each extreme, but always come back home to the calm before you take your next step.

A Note on JR Worsley

Jack Reginald Worsley, known as "JR", is the man credited with bringing Five-Element acupuncture to the Western world. The son of an engineer with an interest in Chinese philosophy, he first worked in a factory before enlisting as an education officer in the British Army during the Second World War. He later became a physiotherapist and an osteopath and began to investigate alternative medical practices, including acupuncture, but it was not until he travelled in Singapore, Taiwan and Korea in the 1950s that he discovered the Five-Element style of acupuncture. He studied and became a "master" and on his return to the UK, founded a school to pass on the teachings he had learnt.

In 1986 I was treated for the first time by a Five Element practitioner in San Francisco, where I was living at that time. I sought treatment because I was feeling very unwell and had just been given a medical diagnosis that suggested my lifespan could be severely shortened. The day after my first treatment I remember feeling profoundly different. I was somewhat perplexed by the striking result of what seemed like just a few random needles but I was excited, intrigued and keen to discover more. My practitioner at the time had been trained by Professor Worsley himself, and suggested I return to the UK to study at Worsley's college in Leamington Spa. By the time I enrolled, Worsley had already trained hundreds of practitioners, many of whom are still working worldwide.

The man was brilliant. He stood miles apart from all other teachers at his college and taught this system of medicine in such a simple way – he used to say a child of five would understand him better than any of us as we struggled to accept the discipline of simplicity. Keeping things simple, experiencing life as it is, is a skill we seem to lose as we grow up and develop our own understanding of our world. My training became an exercise in reawakening my senses and learning to experience my world and the people around me with the same awe and wonder that I had had as a child.

Glossary

Anti-Müllerian Hormone (AMH)
A hormone produced in immature ovary follicles, before they develop to a certain size. It is believed that a low level of AMH therefore means that a woman has fewer follicles that will fully develop into viable ova.

Causative Factor
A term used in Worsley Five-Element acupuncture to describe the element that is the cause of all elemental imbalances in a patient. Having a "causative factor in earth" or "earth CF| means the same as having "a weakness in the earth element".

Clomid
A brand of generic drug, clomiphene citrate, commonly used in treating female infertility to stimulate ovulation.

Donor Insemination
Sperm from a donor is injected into the woman's womb around ovulation.

Egg Donation
A mature egg taken from a donor is mixed with the man's sperm and released into the woman's womb.

Gamete-Intra-Fallopian Transfer (GIFT)
Sperm from the male and eggs taken from the woman's ovaries are

simultaneously placed in one fallopian tube.

Gonadotropin
A hormone produced by the pituitary gland which stimulates the activity of the gonads (ovaries in the female, testicles in the male).

Intra-Cytoplasmic Sperm Injection (ICSI)
An egg in a laboratory dish has a single sperm injected directly into it, and if fertilisation results, the egg is placed in the woman's womb.

Intra-Uterine Insemination (IUI)
A sample of semen from the male partner is examined to find the best-quality sperm which are then injected into the woman's womb around ovulation.

In-Vitro Fertilisation (IVF)
A mature egg and sperm are brought together in a laboratory dish and the fertilised egg is then inserted into the woman's womb.

In-Vitro Maturation (IVM)
Eggs are removed from the woman at an early stage and mature in a laboratory dish. The fertilised egg is then implanted into the woman's womb.

Meridian
In acupuncture or Chinese medicine, this term refers to the pathways along which the body's vital energy flows.

Ovarian Hyperstimulation Syndrome (OHSS)
A medical condition affecting the ovaries of some women who take fertility medication to stimulate egg growth. It can be a potentially serious complication of fertility treatment, particularly IVF.

Reproductive Immunology
A drug treatment to suppress the immune system based on the theory that the body's immune cells might reject the implantation of fertilised eggs. There is no proof of the validity of the theory or the treatment.

Taoism or Daoism
A system of philosophy developed from traditional Chinese religions from the sixth century BC onwards. It is the philosophy that underpins Classical Five-Element acupuncture.

Traditional Chinese Medicine (TCM)
A system of medicine created under Chairman Mao that draws on ancient Chinese traditions as well as those of modern Western science.

Yin and Yang
A concept in Chinese philosophy that describes how duality forms a whole. Yin is characterised as slow, soft, yielding, diffuse, cold, wet or tranquil, and is associated with water, earth, the moon, femininity and nighttime. Yang, by contrast, is fast, hard, solid, focused, hot, dry or aggressive, and is associated with fire, sky, the sun, masculinity and daytime.

Acknowledgements

I am deeply grateful to Clare Conville who encouraged me to write and share my work with patients. Tessa Dunlop and Charlotte Robertson who saw the value of the hidden message in this book and who introduced it to my publishers – Aurea Carpenter and Rebecca Nicolson – who had the vision and courage to make it accessible to a wider audience.

I am eternally grateful to Johnny Childs and Wren Winfield, whose invaluable input, enthusiasm and love are woven into these pages.

Finally I want to thank all of my teachers and my patients who entrusted me with their care and taught me so much.

GERAD KITE is an internationally renowned fertility expert, Acupuncture Master (AcM) and psychotherapist with more than 25 years of clinical experience. In 1993 he started the first NHS acupuncture service at King's College Hospital and in 2005 he opened the Kite Clinic in London, where he heads a team of practitioners performing over 10,000 treatments a year. He is a senior teacher of Worsley Five-Element acupuncture and trains apprentices at his residential training centre in the South of France. He is the author of *Everything You Need You Have* (Short Books, 2016).